公共卫生专业英语教程
English Tutorial for Public Health

主　编 邹华春

副主编 蔡　泳　陈青松

编　者（以姓氏笔画为序）

王冬亮（中山大学）　　　　　　　邹华春（复旦大学）

孔令杰（浙江省卫生健康委员会）　陆少游（中山大学）

卢　雍（贵州医科大学）　　　　　陈青松（广东药科大学）

冯铁建（深圳市疾病预防控制中心）范　颂（西南医科大学）

仲崇科（苏州大学）　　　　　　　范引光（安徽医科大学）

刘斯洋（中山大学）　　　　　　　周　涛（中山大学）

江洪波（广东药科大学）　　　　　孟荟萃（中山大学）

孙力涛（中山大学）　　　　　　　徐明明（中山大学）

孙彩军（中山大学）　　　　　　　蒋亚文（中山大学）

杜向军（中山大学）　　　　　　　褚敏捷（南通大学）

杨淑娟（四川大学）　　　　　　　蔡　泳（上海交通大学医学院附属同仁医院）

学术秘书（以姓氏笔画为序）

王炳懿（中山大学）　　　　　　　付雷雯（中山大学）

人民卫生出版社
·北　京·

版权所有，侵权必究！

图书在版编目（CIP）数据

公共卫生专业英语教程 / 邹华春主编. —北京：
人民卫生出版社，2024.6
ISBN 978-7-117-35691-6

Ⅰ.①公…　Ⅱ.①邹…　Ⅲ.①公共卫生–英语–教材
Ⅳ.①R126.4

中国国家版本馆 CIP 数据核字（2023）第 239990 号

人卫智网　**www.ipmph.com**	医学教育、学术、考试、健康，购书智慧智能综合服务平台	
人卫官网　**www.pmph.com**	人卫官方资讯发布平台	

公共卫生专业英语教程
Gonggong Weisheng Zhuanye Yingyu Jiaocheng

主　　编：邹华春
出版发行：人民卫生出版社（中继线 010-59780011）
地　　址：北京市朝阳区潘家园南里 19 号
邮　　编：100021
E - mail：pmph @ pmph.com
购书热线：010-59787592　010-59787584　010-65264830
印　　刷：北京瑞禾彩色印刷有限公司
经　　销：新华书店
开　　本：787 × 1092　1/16　　印张：11
字　　数：275 千字
版　　次：2024 年 6 月第 1 版
印　　次：2024 年 8 月第 1 次印刷
标准书号：ISBN 978-7-117-35691-6
定　　价：59.00 元
打击盗版举报电话：010-59787491　E-mail：WQ @ pmph.com
质量问题联系电话：010-59787234　E-mail：zhiliang @ pmph.com
数字融合服务电话：4001118166　E-mail：zengzhi @ pmph.com

前　言

在这个全球化的时代，公共卫生问题已经成为全世界人民的共同关注。随着国际的联系与合作愈加紧密，英语成为公共卫生专业交流和合作的重要工具。因此，我们精心编撰了《公共卫生专业英语教程》，旨在帮助公共卫生专业学生和研究人员提升英语水平，更好地掌握国际公共卫生领域最新的研究知识和方法。

本教程共分为十二个单元，分别为公共卫生与预防医学、慢性病流行病学、传染病流行病学、职业与环境卫生学、营养与食品卫生学、妇幼卫生保健学、健康教育学、系统流行病学、重大公共卫生事件及其应对、病原与传染病防控、卫生经济与卫生管理学、循证医学与系统综述。在编写过程中，我们注重理论与实践的结合，每个单元都包含了相关知识和实例，旨在帮助读者更好地理解和应用所学知识。编写本教程时，我们遵循以下原则：①目标导向。以培养学生的公共卫生英语能力为主要目标，全面涵盖公共卫生领域的知识和技能。②学生中心。充分考虑学生的学习需求和兴趣，设计具有启发性、互动性和趣味性的教学内容和活动。③教材权威。汇集公共卫生领域权威专家的研究成果和实践经验，使教材具有权威性和实用性。④跨学科融合。公共卫生是一门跨学科的学科，融合了医学、社会学、经济学、环境科学等学科的知识，以提供全面的视角和深入的理解。⑤前沿性。基于公共卫生研究前沿，面向国际化和全球化教育需求，扩展学生的国际视野。

非常感谢各位编委的支持，他们认真负责、严谨求实的态度，以及扎实宽厚的专业知识保证了本教程的质量。感谢中山大学公共卫生学院（深圳）在本教程编写过程中提供的诸多支持。

我们的共同愿望是吸收目前最新以及最佳的内容，丰富和拓展本教程的科学内涵，更好地服务于我国医学高等教育和人才培养的使命。在本教程的编写过程中，难免存在不足，敬请应用本教程的师生和同道，不吝给予批评和指正。

邹华春

2024 年 2 月

目　录

Contents

Unit 1 Public Health and Preventive Medicine

READING A

PREVIEW

Public health evolved from a narrowly disease-centered to broader population-based, multidisciplinary and multisectoral discipline that is "collective action for sustained improvement of the health of all people". The public health system plays a vital role in the development of health sector and protects the health of people. Globally, most countries are in a period of transition in their public health landscape due to new challenges. Practices in public health at a community-level must be strengthened worldwide. China has robust systems to respond to infectious diseases and is well placed to develop and strengthen community public health systems to tackle non-communicable diseases and health inequalities. Reform, modernization, and investment in a prevention-focused primary care system that integrates with public health services could improve health across the country and ensure that China's trajectory of improving health continues and leaves no one behind. Getting the development and reform right is important to China's social and economic development in the future, and we believe that China's experience in public health may provide many lessons for other countries.

Questions for Discussion

Q 1: What is the significance of community-level public health for disease prevention?

Q 2: What achievements has China made in disease prevention?

Text A

Development and Reform of Public Health in China

The term "public health" has always been vaguely defined. According to Winslow, a leading public health expert, public health is the science and art of preventing disease, prolonging life, and promoting health through the organized efforts and informed choices of society, organizations, public and private communities, and individuals. The United States, the United Kingdom, Australia, the World Health Organization(WHO)/ Western Pacific Region (WPR), and other countries or organizations have identified the basic functions of public health or the scope of basic services that should be delivered by the public health system. Internationally, public health consists of 3 categories of services: population-based public health services, including vector control and population-wide health education; individual-based preventive care, for instance, vaccination, premarital checkup and prenatal care; and individual-based curative care against conditions affecting the health of the public. Public health is closely linked to social and economic development, demographic structure, disease pattern and disease burden and existing administrative system. These factors vary considerably from country to country and region to region.

The public health system plays a vital role in the development of the health sector in China and improves the health of the Chinese people. Given that the history and structure of China's public health system has its own characteristics, it is worth looking at the development of public health in China. It is **crucial** to understand why and how China has achieved such a success, as this may be useful to other countries.

Public health in China has gone through four key phases: an initial phase centered on prevention, a deviant phase that focused more on treatment and less on prevention, a recovery phase after the SARS (severe **acute** respiratory **syndrome**) crisis, and a new phase towards equity and people-centeredness. In the most recent phase, the National Basic Public Health Service Program (NBPHSP) was **implemented** to address the threat of non-communicable diseases (NCDs) and some initial results were achieved.

The development of public health in China has been marked by both unique Chinese wisdom, remarkable achievements and twists and turns. Prevention is the main focus. Institutional flexibility, multi-agency collaboration, mass mobilization, and social participation were the main lessons learned from the early days of public health. Although China's public health system has shown great resilience since the 1980s, this may be due to the government's continued commitment to social development and people's livelihoods, as well as its flexible governance.

Since the outbreak of SARS in 2002, health-care **reform** in China has been **squarely** focused on community-level capacity building, in contrast to countries with less-than-ideal community **surveillance** systems.

Disease control and prevention based on community mobilization are **fundamental** in China. Back in the 1950s, the Chinese government initiated its all-in-all Patriotic Health Campaign, and has been keeping the pace for the intervening decades, increasing life expectancy from 35 years in 1949 to 77 years in 2019. Many diseases have been effectively controlled. In addition to the **eradication** of **smallpox** and **elimination** of **polio**, following the world's lead, China has eliminated or almost eliminated diseases such as **malaria**, **leprosy**, **filariasis**, and **schistosomiasis**. Most importantly, this feat has been accomplished by **strengthening** capacity and practice at the community level. In the early stages, the organizational mechanism of the system was the establishment of so-called stratified epidemic prevention stations, ranging from provincial to local to county levels. The system worked well with the National Immunization Program, which began in the late 1970s and allowed for effective control of vaccine-preventable diseases, especially for infants and children. However, we realized that our national-level scientific and technical support system was not sufficient to support the **entire enterprise**.

To address this core need, a system similar to that of the US Center for Disease Control and Prevention (CDC) -known as the China CDC -was established in 2002, just before the SARS **outbreak**. To establish this new system, a national research organization, the Chinese Academy of Preventive Medicine, was transformed into the China CDC. Regional stations were retained and renamed as local CDCs, from provincial to local to county levels, unlike the US CDC system. Since then, China's four-level CDC system has been well built with comprehensive capacity and large **workforce**.

In the 2010s, in order to achieve a well-off society, the Chinese government pays unprecedented attention to the health sector, which brings a new wave of development opportunities for public health such as the continuation of the priority of NBPHSP. The development and reform of public health in China is based on its national condition, and has accumulated a wealth of experience, as well as facing many common worldwide challenges. Getting this development and reform right is important for China's social and economic development in the future, and China's experience in public health may provide many lessons for other countries.

The "Healthy China 2030" initiative, which began in 2016, promotes the **integration** of prevention and clinical medicine. Prevention is regarded as the most effective measure for disease control. Capacity building at the community level is an ongoing **priority** in Healthy China 2030. In order to achieve Healthy China 2030 goals, political will is essential to **adequate** financial support and **coordination** with **stakeholders** and the public. Community-level clinics and county-level CDCs are also encouraged to **collaborate** in the management of non-communicable diseases. Private sector organizations and non-governmental organizations are encouraged to participate in health care reform at the community level. **Nevertheless**, there is considerable work to do. For example, rabies remains a problem in China, which is not commensurate with the country's level of development. With such a large, **geographically diverse** country with inequality in economic development, diseases such as rabies will need to be addressed in the future. One Health concepts and practices are needed for any measure of success. There are a number of zoonotic diseases that need to be managed through coordination between the health and agricultural sectors, particularly in rural areas where there are gaps in public health practices at the community level. **Tobacco** use remains a huge problem in China, and community-level public health practice should be called upon to play a key role for long-term solutions.

Globally, most countries are in a period of transition in their public health landscape due to common new challenges. The development and reform of public health in China needs to be further deepened. Firstly, the accelerating aging population has put a number of countries at a considerable disadvantage in terms of health care reform. Developing countries are experiencing a much more rapid aging process than rich countries, and China is the fastest one in the coming decades. This is a serious potential risk to the financial sustainability of China's health sector in a broader sense. Furthermore, lower fertility intentions may exacerbate the risk. It is similar to the situation in the Next Eleven (Next-11) countries where healthcare expenditure has risen sharply, due to a higher proportion of the elderly and lower fertility rates. Secondly, NCDs are recognized as the key health challenge worldwide, and have emerged as the number one health threat in China. Unlike infectious diseases which have a relatively short acute phase and a short cure time, NCDs will place a huge and long-term burden on patients and society. Moreover, the prevalence of NCDs is disproportionately high among older people, some of whom often have more than one NCD. The emerging NCDs burden coupled with an aging population means that sustainability challenges in the public health system will be very serious, even in the richest Organization for Economic Co-operation and Development countries. Thirdly, social and economic transformation have accelerated urbanization and lifestyle changes, leading to many risk factors such as obesity, sedentary lifestyles, stress, tobacco/alcohol/other substances abuse, and exposure to pollution. The incidence of NCDs is also rising due to these individual or environmental factors. Fourthly, globalization has accelerated the spread of infectious diseases, imposing challenges to public health. Many countries, including China, are facing the dual burden of NCDs and infectious diseases at the same time.

In a nutshell, the evolution and reform of China's public health is based on its national condition. During the process, China accumulates rich experience but also faces many common worldwide challenges which may be even more pronounced in China.

Public health in China needs to focus on prevention, strengthen multi-agency coordination mechanism, and improve the quality of public health services in the future. However, it is expected that the government's continuous attention to the health sector and its stable macro environment will be greatly helpful to address those challenges. Getting this development and reform right is important to China's social and economic development in the future. China's experience in public health may provide many lessons for other countries.

Practices in public health at a community-level must be strengthened worldwide. Disease knows no borders and we should work together to **tackle** the common enemies of mankind. China needs the world and vice versa.

Words and Expressions

crucial 至关重要的

*For executive function and social skills, existing research leans against the **crucial** causal position but is insufficient to differentiate the other 2.*

acute 急性的

*Avoidance and treatment of hypoxemia is a cornerstone of **acute** resuscitation and yet the optimal approach to oxygen therapy in the acute care setting is uncertain.*

syndrome 综合征

*The shape of the face is affected in 30%-40% of known genetic **syndromes**.*

implement 实施

*All nurses have responsibilities to enculturate evidence-based practice (EBP) and translate and **implement** research findings into nursing care, practices, and procedures.*

reform　改革

*Major health policy creation or changes, including governmental and private policies affecting health care delivery, are based on health care **reform(s)**.*

squarely　直接地

*They placed the blame **squarely** on the president.*

surveillance　监视,监测

*Two important measurements for the evaluation of a public health **surveillance** system are sensitivity and predictive value positive (PVP).*

fundamental　基本的,关键的

*Efforts are underway to heighten nurses' awareness of values that motivate **fundamental** care and thereby increase their attention to effective provision of **fundamental** care.*

eradication　根除

*Because of the success of global measles control programs, the World Health Organization (WHO), along with its partner agencies, is once again considering the possibility of setting a target date for measles **eradication**.*

smallpox　天花

*Widespread vaccination programs led to the global eradication of **smallpox**, which was certified by the World Health Organization (WHO), and, since 1978, there has been no case of **smallpox** anywhere in the world.*

elimination　消除

*Since 2005, malaria cases have been declining globally with many countries having eliminated malaria and several other countries heading towards malaria **elimination**.*

polio　脊髓灰质炎

*The Global **Polio** Eradication Initiative since 1988 has seen the impact of poliovirus decline from frequent global epidemics in the early 1900s to being now only endemic in two countries today.*

malaria　疟疾

*Important strides have been made within the past decade toward **malaria** elimination in many regions, and with this progress, the feasibility of eradication is once again under discussion.*

leprosy　麻风病

***Leprosy** is often not suspected because it is no longer emphasized in the medical curricula.*

filariasis　丝虫病

***Filariases** are infections caused by distinct species of nematodes.*

schistosomiasis　血吸虫病

*Despite accelerating progress towards **schistosomiasis** control in sub-Saharan Africa, several age groups have been eclipsed by current treatment and monitoring strategies that mainly focus on school-aged children.*

strengthen　加强,强化

*Supraspinatus **strengthening** is an important part of shoulder rehabilitation programs.*

entire　全部的,完全的

*When dysplasia is identified in a gallbladder, many experts recommend submission of the **entire*** *gallbladder for histologic examination.*

enterprise 企业，事业单位

*Enterprise imaging governance is an emerging need in health **enterprises** today.*

outbreak 暴发

*A main goal of syndromic surveillance systems is to detect outbreaks rapidly and the number of studies evaluating **outbreak** detection has increased recently.*

workforce 全体员工，劳动力

*A suitably skilled **workforce** that is of an appropriate size is essential for the provision of healthcare services.*

integration 整合，一体化

*This **integration** process requires the appropriate allocation of cognitive resources to both the gesture and speech modalities.*

priority 优先，优先事项

*Nurses participated in organizational and societal level **priority** setting through discussion about the **priorities**.*

adequate 足够的，适当的

*Detailed knowledge about the different types of impingement and the underlying causes is essential to provide **adequate** treatment.*

coordination 协调

*Clearly identified professionals who are appointed for care **coordination** are invaluable for ensuring efficient coordination of health care services.*

stakeholder 利益相关者，有权益关系者

*Health care innovations tailored to **stakeholder** context are more readily adopted.*

collaborate 合作

*Coalitions implementing health promotion initiatives are composed of organizations that **collaborate** with one another.*

nevertheless 尽管如此

***Nevertheless**, many researchers have tried to solve these problems, and it is hoped that transgenic animals in combination with newer immunosuppressive treatment will make xenotransplantation a realistic possibility.*

geographically 在地理上

*Overview of **geographically** explicit momentary assessment research, applied to the study of mental health and well-being, which allows for cross-validation, extension, and enrichment of research on place and health.*

diverse 各种各样的，不同的

*A DNA-encoded chemical library (DECL) is built with combinatorial chemistry, which works by bringing chemical fragments together to generate **diverse** structures.*

tobacco 烟草

*The oral cavities of **tobacco** smokers and users of smokeless **tobacco** products are exposed to high concentrations of nicotine.*

tackle　处理，解决

*Immune cell-based therapies are emerging as a promising tool to **tackle** malignancies, both solid tumors and selected hematological tumors.*

Language Points

infectious diseases　感染性疾病

A disease (such as influenza, malaria, meningitis, rabies, or tetanus) caused by the entrance into the body of pathogenic agents or microorganisms (such as bacteria, viruses, protozoans, or fungi) which grow and multiply there. Including communicable diseases and non-communicable diseases.

***Infectious diseases** have for centuries ranked with wars and famine as major challenges to human progress and survival.*

communicable diseases　传染病

An infectious disease (as cholera, hepatitis, influenza, malaria, measles, or tuberculosis) that is transmissible by contact with infected individuals or their bodily discharges or fluids (as respiratory droplets, blood, or semen), by contact with contaminated surfaces or objects, by ingestion of contaminated food or water, or by direct or indirect contact with disease vectors (as mosquitoes, fleas, or mice).

*The terms **communicable disease** and contagious disease are often used interchangeably. However, communicable diseases such as malaria or schistosomiasis that are spread by contact with disease vectors are not typically considered to be "contagious" diseases since they cannot be spread from direct contact with another person.*

zoonotic diseases　人畜共患病

Zoonotic diseases are defined by the World Health Organization as, "those diseases and infections naturally transmitted between man and other vertebrate animals."

Global economics and advances in technolgy have contributed to the emergence or re-emergence of infectious diseases and to the spread of zoonotic diseases that would otherwise have been confined to local areas.

EXERCISES

Task 1: Vocabulary Application

Fill in the blanks with the words given below. Change the form where necessary.

> **reform; coordinate; pandemic; strengthen; elimination; mortality; threat; chronic; decade; ecological**

1. Particularly, leadership in district hospitals needs to _____ in order to decrease the burden of perinatal _____ .

2. The social and _____ changes accompanying the Anthropocene（人类纪）require

changes in how _____ are anticipated, conceived, and managed.

3. Hepatitis C infection is a serious public health _____ , and the World Health Organization has recommended the _____ of public health threats from viral hepatitis, including hepatitis C, by 2030.

4. The 2016 President's Cancer Panel Connected Health report calls for thoroughly characterizing the team structures and processes involved in _____ care for people with _____ conditions.

5. During the last _____ , policy makers in a large number of countries have attempted various _____ of their health care systems.

Task 2: Writing

For this part, you are allowed 30 minutes to write a composition on the topic Epidemics. You should write at least 120 words, and base your composition on the outline below:

1) Epidemics can be seen everywhere in our lives.

2) What harm will epidemics bring?

3) What measures should we take to control epidemics?

Task 3: Oral Presentation

Mankind has a wealth of experience in combating pandemics. Combining epidemiological knowledge, give an example about pandemics and describe the corresponding epidemic prevention measures from the perspective of public health.

READING B

PREVIEW

Public health, when working well, is invisible. However, when a public health system is chronically underfunded, understaffed, undertrained, and undersupported, the consequences are immense and visible. The pandemic of emerging infectious diseases has made our nation more aware than ever the important role public health plays in surveillance and screening to contain outbreaks, and the distribution of vaccines and other essential resources to control them. Although public health education in general is expanding, it is doing so at a slower pace than many other health science disciplines. The multidisciplinary and multisectoral nature of public health may pose a challenge to organizing public health education. Currently, most clinical physicians in China do not receive public health training, and most public health professionals responsible for disease control are not equipped with sufficient clinical skills. Existing undergraduate and graduate curricula for the preventive medicine may unintentionally widen the gap between public health and clinical medicine. It is urgently needed to strengthen preventive medicine curriculum in training programs for clinical medical students in the new era.

Questions for Discussion

Q1: How to bridge the gaps between clinical medicine and public health for disease control in China?

Q2: Why do graduates of top preventive medicine programs show little interest in working at CDCs?

Text B

Public Health and Preventive Medicine Education in China: Things to Consider
Defining Public Health

Public health has evolved, so has the definition of public health. Common to most definitions is a sense of the general public interest, a focus on the broader determinants of health, and a desire to improve the health of the entire population. Earlier definitions also made **explicit** reference to the administration of health-care services. The plethora of definitions suggests the need for a short and **succinct** definition of public health that is both broad in scope and of wide appeal. In fact, public health evolved from a narrowly disease-centered to a broader population-based, multidisciplinary and multisectoral **discipline** that is "collective action for sustained improvement of the health of all people". It requires contributions from various disciplines: sociologists, economists, politicians, environmentalists, epidemiologists, statisticians, clinicians, etc.

Public Health and Preventive Medicine in China

The difference between preventive medicine and public health has not been well recognized in most countries, including China. From the 1950s to the 1970s, China's model of public health education was imported from the former Soviet Union, with an emphasis on **sanitation** and **hygiene**. During this era, many medical universities and colleges established departments of hygiene, or as it was later called, preventive medicine. Public health education mainly consisted of five core disciplines: food and nutrition, environmental health, occupational health, radiation health, and school health. Beginning in the 1980s, departments of preventive medicine began to establish schools of public health. New disciplines based on western models were also established, including epidemiology, health statistics, social medicine, and health policy and management.

Based on the technical developments in epidemiology in the middle of the last century, public health has been dominated by the **quantitative** sciences at the expense of other public health sciences. Preventive medicine is often treated as a specialty of medicine, and therefore has clinical training as its foundation, with additional training in public health. According to its educational curriculum, China does treat preventive medicine as a specialty of medicine. Most undergraduate preventive medicine programs in China require five years of predominantly clinical and basic science training: four years of basic health science and curative medicine, and one year of public health (e.g. epidemiology, biostatistics, occupational health, environmental health, etc.). Afterwards, the students received their medical degrees.

Disease Control System Reforms Potentially Widen the Gap between Public Health and Clinical Medicine

In 2002, the outbreak and spread of SARS drew great attention to the field of public health and the prevention of infectious disease. China established the Chinese Center for Disease Control and Prevention (CDC) in 2002, and divided each Hygiene and Anti-Epidemic Stations

(HAES) at various levels into two separate units: the local CDC and the Health Inspection Unit (HIU). The HIU is the law enforcement unit that ensures various activities, such as food production, comply with national health standards. Meanwhile, many universities or medical schools established Schools of Public Health. Consequently, preventive medicine has become **synonymous** with public health in China, and the two terms are used interchangeably.

Drastic change of **regulations** on the **eligibility** of medical practitioners **unintentionally** distanced preventive medicine from clinical medicine and potentially widened the gap between public health and clinical medicine. The Law on Licensed Doctors of the People's Republic of China implemented in 1999, which **stipulated** the qualification of health professionals working in the field of clinical medicine, disease prevention, and health promotion. A supplemental regulation on the eligibility for national medical professional exams further reiterated that only graduates with a clinical medicine degree were eligible to take the medical board examination and engage in clinical medicine after fifteen years (2014). It profoundly affected preventive medicine graduates' career development. Since then, preventive medicine graduates have not been able to practice clinical medicine. Nor could they practice in the division of infectious diseases at hospitals where they previously sought employment. Preventive medicine graduates cannot practice curative medicine, which generates a disconnection between the curriculum and the practice.

Fundamental Challenges on Human Resources for Disease Control in China

The fundamental challenge for the CDCs is the lack of qualified personnel with both clinical and public health training. Existing undergraduate preventive medicine programs only provide students with one to two years of clinical training, which is not sufficient for them to acquire adequate clinical experience to **tackle communicable** and **non-communicable diseases** at the individual and community levels. Furthermore, education for public health students in China lags behind due to outdated curricula and teaching materials, **excessive** focus on teaching biomedical sciences, insufficient or low-quality practical training in the public health sector. Most students choose to start work immediately after graduation, with only a minority deciding to pursue further studies. Although public health education in general is expanding, it is doing so at a slower pace than many other health science disciplines. At one of the most competitive universities in China, the number of **doctorate students** admitted into public health and preventive medicine programs increased by only 5.3% from 2008 to 2011, which was **substantially** lower than the average 14.1% increase across all disciplines at universities.

The number of master graduates working at the CDCs is significantly lower than the number employed in hospitals. Nearly 35% of the graduates are doing **administrative** or **logistical** work unrelated to their **specializations**. Moreover, a large number of the graduates are employed by provincial-or municipal-level institutions, which results in the relatively low educational level in **rudimentary** CDCs. Many students are often persuaded or assigned to study public health. According to a nationwide survey of 1197 undergraduate public health students, those who chose to study public health as their first preference only accounted for 26.9% of the entire surveyed students, which starkly contrasts against the preferences for students who chose to study medicine (75.0%). With a large proportion of students dissatisfied with their major, these students are more likely to find a job that is not related to health sciences. The survey also found that about one in five public health students were unwilling to find a job in public health after graduation.

Salary is one of the most important factors for job seekers. Along with healthcare reform, the income of hospital medical staff has increased. Nevertheless, due to the nature of the public institutions, CDCs pay relatively low salaries based on standard and performance. Graduates may earn more in hospitals, colleges, and enterprises than in the CDCs or other public health-related institutions, which may be one of the reasons that prevent them from working in disease prevention-related institutions. The initial salary of the master's graduates varied across administrative levels. The study showed that only 30.9% of graduates earned more than CNY 6,000 per month. Due to this reason, the satisfaction rate and work ethic of CDC staff **inevitably** suffer.

Strengthen Preventive Medicine for Disease Control in China

It is **imperative** to reform preventive medicine training to strengthen the links between public health and clinical medicine. Firstly, the curriculum of clinical medicine for undergraduate preventive medicine programs should be strengthened. Undergraduate programs in preventive medicine should have clinical training similar to that of clinical medicine to ensure that preventive medicine undergraduates receive adequate training in clinical medicine. The government should enhance **residency** training programs on preventive medicine and rectify the eligibility regulation to allow preventive medicine graduates to obtain a certificate to practice clinical medicine in the field where public health interventions play a significant role in reducing the disease burden, such as infectious diseases, non-communicable diseases, injuries, and maternal and child health.

Secondly, the training programs should **incorporate** more diverse curricula on public health. The core course should include basic knowledge in these areas: epidemiology, biostatistics, health policy, management, and economics (health services administration); social and behavioral sciences (medical sociology, health education, health promotion, behavior change); and environmental health. These are internationally recognized as the five core areas of public health, which are consistent with the three domains of public health practice, and with curriculum proposed by the Associations of School of Public Health in the USA and Europe. The training programs should also provide more intensive clinical training to meet the increasing demand for **interdisciplinary** skills in disease control.

Finally, it is critical to provide clinical settings for preventive medicine **physicians** to sharpen their clinical skills for disease control. Hospital beds should be allocated for public health physicians to manage inpatients as well and to implement the responsibilities and requirements of public health physicians for patient management. In brief, public health physicians are required to participate in the whole process of patient reception, diagnosis and treatment, operation, medical record writing and follow-up. In the process of clinical practice, public health physicians should attend clinical lectures, teaching rounds and case analysis according to the training plans; so that they could systematically master the clinical knowledge and applications, and achieve certain professional ability to deal with clinical affairs.

Conclusion

The multidisciplinary and multisectoral nature of public health may **pose a challenge to** organizing public health education. Existing undergraduate and graduate curricula for preventive medicine may unintentionally widen the gap between public health and clinical medicine. Enhancing clinical skills, amending the Law on Licensed Doctors of the People′s Republic of China, and expanding the public health curriculum for preventive medicine graduates can better equip professionals to address both global and national health challenges.

Words and Expressions

explicit 明确的

*Parents and teachers can help children by providing **explicit** instruction regarding the mind as a learning machine.*

succinct 简明的

*The book gives an admirably **succinct** account of the technology and its history.*

sanitation 环境卫生；卫生设备和系统

*Many illnesses are the result of inadequate **sanitation**.*

hygiene 卫生

*The government has introduced some tough new laws on food **hygiene**.*

quantitative 定量性的；量化的

*The organizers of the experiment concluded that far fewer students were achieving at high levels on critical thinking than they were doing for written communication or **quantitative** literacy.*

synonymous 同义的；等同于……的

*Wealth is not necessarily **synonymous** with happiness.*

regulation 章程；规章制度

*The European Union has proposed new **regulations** to control the hours worked by its employees.*

eligibility 资格

*The government has altered the rules governing **eligibility** for unemployment benefit.*

unintentionally 无意中

*They had **unintentionally** provided wrong information.*

stipulate 规定；明确要求

*Some jurisdictions permit individuals to waive their right to contest a hearing and instead **stipulate** to civil commitment.*

tackle 解决

*The first reason to **tackle** these problems is to save children's lives.*

excessive 过度的

*Democracy is incompatible with **excessive**, bureaucratic regimentation of social life.*

substantially　大量地，可观地

*Salaries and associated costs have risen **substantially**.*

administrative　管理的；行政的

*I spend a lot of my time on **administrative** duties.*

logistical　后勤的

*She described the distribution of food and medical supplies as a **logistical** nightmare.*

rudimentary　初级的；基本的

*They were given only **rudimentary** training in the job.*

inevitably　不可避免地

*The result will **inevitably** fuel speculation about the Prime Minister's future.*

imperative　重要紧急的；迫切的

*It is **imperative** to continue the treatment for at least two months.*

residency　高级专科住院医生实习期

*On Improving the Capability of Standardized Training **Residency** in Internal Intensive Medicine.*

incorporate　合并；包含

*When we acquire new information, the brain automatically tries to **incorporate** it within existing information by forming associations.*

interdisciplinary　多学科的；跨学科的

*Australian Chinese study is a kind of **interdisciplinary** research on Chinese problems.*

physician　医师；（尤指）内科医生

*I'm a practicing **physician** trying to help people here and now.*

detrimental　有害的；不利的

*Poor eating habits are **detrimental** to health.*

Language Points

bridge the gap　消除隔阂；弥合差距

to have qualities of two different groups or things

*His work **bridges the gap** between popular fiction and serious literature.*

notifiable infectious diseases　法定传染病

Currently, 41 infectious diseases are notifiable in China, classified as Class A, Class B and Class C according to their epidemic levels and potential population threats. Class A and Class B (total 30 diseases) represent categories of diseases with high risk of outbreaks or that are likely to result in rapid spread once an outbreak occurs. Mortality and morbidity related to group A and B diseases are reported and published by the National Health Commission of the People's Republic of China on a monthly basis. Class C diseases are less infectious and, when outbreaks occur, are epidemiologically less severe. They are required to be reported only when outbreaks occur.

*We performed a descriptive study of notifiable infectious diseases among foreigners reported from 2004 to 2017 in China using data from the Chinese National **Notifiable Infectious Disease** Reporting System (NNIDRIS).*

pose a challenge to 给……带来挑战

*Polio **poses a** particular **challenge to** countries with unstable politics and weak health systems.*

undergraduate 大学本科生

a student who is studying for their first degree at a college or university

postgraduate 研究生

a student who has already received one degree and is studying at a university for a more advanced degree

*We thank our colleagues, collaborators, **postgraduate** and **undergraduate** students who have contributed to, motivated and inspired our research activities in this field.*

Center for Disease Control and Prevention (CDC) 疾病预防控制中心

Chinese Center for Disease Control and Prevention (briefly as China CDC) is a governmental and national-level technical organization specialized on disease control and prevention and public health. Its mission is to create a safe and healthy environment, maintain social stability, ensure national security and promote the health of people through prevention and control of disease, injury and disability. Devoted itself to disease control and prevention, it sticks to relying on scientific research and values talent as a fundamental element.

***CDC** conducts critical science and provides health information that protects our nation against expensive and dangerous health threats, and responds when these arise.*

EXERCISES

Task 1: Vocabulary Application

Fill in the blanks with the words given below. Change the form where necessary.

> **occupational; hygiene; infectious; curriculum; certification; surveillance; complement; residency; medical record; adoption**

1. As a result of the _____ disease pandemic, commercial hand _____ products have become scarce and World Health Organization (WHO) alcohol-based hand rub formulations containing ethanol or isopropanol are being produced for hospitals worldwide.

2. In Germany, _____ skin diseases have topped the annual list of suspected work-related diseases for years.

3. With the evolution of digital media, areas such as public health are adding new platforms to _____ traditional systems of epidemiological _____.

4. In the first decades of the 21st century, a major transition is underway in documentation of patient-related data in clinical settings with the rapid acceleration of the <u>adoption</u> of electronic _____ .

5. To determine which methods best prepare psychiatry residents for the _____ exam, and ultimately for practice, to facilitate appropriate _____ program _____

changes.

Task 2: Writing

The Lancet is collecting ideas from preventive medicine students about public health. For this part, you are allowed to write a letter to the Editor of the Lancet to express your views on the importance of public health system reform. You should write at least 150 words but no more than 300 words.

Task 3: Oral Presentation

Debate involves an individual or a team of students working to effectively convince a judge that their side of a resolution or topic is, as a general principle, more valid. Students in debate come to thoroughly understand both sides of an issue, having researched each extensively, and learn to think critically about every argument that could be made on each side.

For this part, please hold a debate with the topic "Is it necessary for clinicians to receive public health training?".

Learning Garden

Concept of the Essential Public Health Functions

Public health refers to the science and art of preventing disease, prolonging life and promoting, protecting and improving health through organized efforts of society. The essential public health functions (EPHFs) are generally regarded as a fundamental and indispensable set of collective actions under the responsibility of the State which are needed to meet public health goals, including the attainment and maintenance of the highest level of population health possible within given resources. The list of and the way of operationalizing EPHFs are dependent on societal and health contexts in a country or region and the EPHFs are interconnected and interdependent.

A list of common and fundamental public health functions was developed through a crosswalk and analysis of different authoritative lists of EPHFs. This consolidated list is presented to facilitate further global discussion on the application of EPHFs, rather than as an agreed global framework.

A list of public health functions identified as common and fundamental based on a crosswalk analysis of essential public health functions lists:

1. Monitoring and evaluating the population's health status, health service utilization and surveillance of risk factors and threats to health

2. Public health emergency management

3. Assuring effective public health governance, regulation and legislation

4. Supporting efficient and effective health systems and multisectoral planning, financing and management for population health

5. Protecting populations against health threats, including environment and occupational hazards, communicable disease threats, food safety, chemical and radiation hazards

6. Promoting prevention and early detection of diseases, including noncommunicable and communicable diseases

7. Promoting health and well-being and actions to address the wider determinants of health and inequity

8. Ensuring community engagement, participation and social mobilization for health and well-being

9. Ensuring adequate quantity and quality of public health workforce

10. Assuring quality of and access to health services

11. Advancing public health research

12. Ensuring equitable access to and rational use of essential medicines and other health technologies

（邹华春）

Unit 2　Epidemiology of Chronic Diseases

READING A

PREVIEW

Chronic diseases are defined broadly as conditions that last one year or more and require ongoing medical attention or limit activities of daily living or both. Chronic diseases such as cardiovascular disease, cancer, respiratory disease, and diabetes are the leading causes of death. Chronic diseases have major adverse effects on the quality of life of affected individuals, cause premature death, and create large adverse economic effects on families, communities and societies in general. Although common and costly, many chronic diseases are also preventable. Chronic diseases do not occur at random and usually have causal risk and preventive factors that can be found. Many chronic diseases are caused by a short list of risk behaviors including tobacco use, unhealthy diet, physical inactivity, and harmful use of alcohol. If these major risk factors were eliminated, about three-quarters of heart disease, strokes, type 2 diabetes and 40% of cancers could be prevented.

Questions for Discussion

Q1: What are the differences between non-communicable diseases and communicable diseases?

Q2: What are the main strategies and actions for preventing and controlling non-communicable diseases?

Text A

Risk Factors and Prevention of Non-communicable Diseases

Noncommunicable diseases (NCDs), also known as chronic diseases, tend to be of long duration and are the result of a combination of **genetic**, **physiological**, environmental, and behavioral factors. The main types of NCDs are cardiovascular diseases (e.g., heart attacks and stroke), cancers, **chronic respiratory diseases** (e.g., chronic obstructive pulmonary disease and asthma), and diabetes. NCDs are usually characterized by **insidious onset** and long duration (more than three months from diagnosis). Additionally, they often lack clear evidence of biological causes by infectious agents and are not transmitted from person to person.

NCDs are now the leading cause of death and **disability** worldwide. Most chronic illnesses are unable to heal and are generally difficult to be cured completely. Some can be immediately life-threatening, such as heart disease and stroke. Others linger over time and need intensive management, such as diabetes. The **epidemic** of NCDs has posed devastating health **consequences** for individuals, families, and communities, and has been threatening to overwhelm the health systems. Cardiovascular diseases, cancer, respiratory diseases, and diabetes are among the major ones that endanger human health, decrease people's life quality, and are collectively responsible for almost 70% of all deaths worldwide. Almost three-quarters of all NCD deaths, and 82% of the 16 million people who died prematurely, or before age 70, occur in low-and middle-income countries. In China, as estimated, the loss of all-cause **disability-adjusted life years (DALYs)** in 2010 was 320 million person-years, of which NCDs accounted for 77%. The top five were cardiovascular disease, cancer, musculoskeletal disorders, mental and behavioral disorders, and chronic respiratory diseases.

As mentioned previously, due to the prolonged duration of chronic diseases and their unknown **etiology**, NCDs lead to long-term medical costs, permanent economic stress for individuals, families, societies, and countries. Therefore, the **socioeconomic** costs associated with NCDs make the prevention and control of these diseases a major development imperative for the 21st century.

Distribution of NCDs

NCDs have their specific features of time, population, and regional distribution. For instance, due to their long duration, the **prevalence** of chronic diseases has surged over time and has not yet slowed down. Prevalence also varies by country and gender. For some reason, in high-income countries, lung cancer causes more deaths among men, while deaths from breast cancer are more common among women. In contrast, in Africa, **cervical** cancer is the leading cancer causing a high proportion of deaths among women. However, the prevalence of NCDs is increasing rapidly in both high-income and low-income countries. The explanation for this increase is not only the rise of risk factors but also a change in diagnostic criteria.

Main Risk Factors

Diseases and other health-related events do not occur at random and usually have causal risk and preventive factors that can be found. The rise of NCDs is driven by four main risk factors: tobacco use, physical inactivity, harmful use of alcohol, and unhealthy diet.

Tobacco Use

Tobacco has been demonstrated to contain at least 250 identified harmful substances and more than 50 **carcinogens**. About one-sixth of **mortality** from NCDs can be attributed to tobacco as an exposure factor. Almost six million people die from tobacco use each year, both from direct tobacco use and second-hand smoking. By 2020, this number increased to 7.5 million, accounting for 10% of all deaths. Smoking has been estimated to be responsible for about 71% of lung cancer, 42% of chronic respiratory disease, and nearly 10% of cardiovascular disease. However, tobacco consumption continues to increase rapidly in low-income and middle-income countries. To promote health, WHO recommended the adoption of the

MPOWER tobacco control strategy in 2008, which includes monitoring tobacco use, protecting people against tobacco harms, providing smoking cessation assistance, warning about the harms of tobacco, banning advertising, and raising taxes, etc.

Physical Inactivity

The lack of physical activity is associated with a 20% to 30% increased risk of all-cause mortality. Regular and moderate physical activity facilitates energy balance, controls weight, builds muscle, and promotes cardiorespiratory fitness. Previous studies have demonstrated that moderate exercise reduces the risk of cardiovascular disease, diabetes, cancer, and depression. On the contrary, a **sedentary** lifestyle has been demonstrated to be a risk of diabetes and rectal cancer.

Harmful Use of Alcohol

Alcohol abuse is a major risk factor for **premature** death and disability by increasing the risk of hypertension, stroke, and other diseases. Each year, excessive alcohol abuse causes 3.3 million deaths (5.9% of all deaths) worldwide. The problem is also serious among young people: about a quarter of deaths in the 20-39 age group are caused by alcohol abuse.

Unhealthy Diet

Adequate fruit and vegetable consumption reduces the risk of cardiovascular, diseases, stomach cancer, and colorectal cancer. While on the contrary, an unhealthy diet causes at least 14 million deaths each year. Most people consume far more salt than the level recommended by WHO for disease prevention (less than five grams of salt per person per day). High salt consumption is an important cause of high blood pressure, posing a risk for cardiovascular disease. Similarly, high consumption of **saturated fats** and **trans-fatty acids** has been linked to heart disease.

Prevention

The most frequently employed prevention strategies are population strategies and high-risk strategies.

Population strategies represent prevention approaches that target the whole population or large population subgroups. Population strategies are used where there is a mass exposure to risk, even if that risk is at a low level. Therefore, the greatest benefit will be achieved by the community by shifting the whole distribution curve. The primary methods commonly used are health education, health promotion, and community interventions. Examples of these approaches are the iodization household salt, the compulsory use of car seat belts, and increasing taxes on tobacco products, etc.

In comparison, high-risk prevention strategies target individuals or groups that made the major contribution to the **incidence** rate, usually due to an exposure to the presence of modifiable risk factors known to have a causal effect on the disease. Once identified, interventions are targeted to these individuals or groups to modify their risk of disease or illness.

Both of the two intervention strategies have their **priorities** and specificities and, in reality, need to be combined in the prevention and control of NCDs.

Three Levels of Prevention

Primary Prevention

Primary prevention aims to prevent a disease or injury before it ever occurs. For NCDs, primary prevention is usually accomplished by preventing exposure to risk factors from hazards that cause disease or injury before they occur. It is one of the fundamental measures to prevent the occurrence of chronic diseases. Generally, it contains two types: health promotion and specific prevention. Example of primary prevention includes education about healthy habits (e.g. eating well, exercising regularly, not smoking) and safety consciousness.

Secondary Prevention

Secondary prevention aims to reduce the impact of a disease or injury that has already occurred. It typically contains early **detection**, early diagnosis, and early treatment, with the goal of stopping or slowing the progression of the disease once it has occurred. Common measures include regular examinations and **screening** tests, which enable the timely detection of people undergoing the early onset of the disease and improve **prognosis** and prolong **survival time**. The frequency of the screen can be determined by demographical characteristics of the disease such as age, gender, occupation, etc.

Tertiary Prevention

Tertiary prevention focuses on softening the impact of an ongoing illness or injury that has lasting effects. It is the prevention of disability and the promotion of physiological recovery to improve a patient's function capacity, quality of life, **life expectancy**, as well as reduce mortality.

Words and Expressions

cardiovascular　心血管的

*Coronary heart disease (CHD) is the most **cardiovascular** disease which damaged people's health these days.*

respiratory　呼吸的

*Sales of **respiratory** masks, spurred by swine flu, demand boosted results.*

diabetes　糖尿病

*People with high blood pressure are especially vulnerable to **diabetes**.*

preventive　预防的, 防备的

*The authors do not address **preventive** interventions that occur outside the doctor's office.*

stroke　卒中

*She has, in the past couple of years, suffered a **stroke** and had heart surgery.*

genetic　基因的, 遗传学的

*The disease has a **genetic** element.*

physiological　生理的, 生理功能的

*We can get hormone levels, **physiological** data, disease status.*

infectious　传染的, 传染性的

*Flu is highly **infectious***.

insidious　阴险的；隐伏的

*Narcotics addiction is **insidious***.

onset　开始，发作

*Most of the passes have been closed with the **onset** of winter.*

disability　残疾，缺陷

***Disability** is a physical limitation on people's life.*

epidemic　流行病，传染病

*Today, doctors are fearing a worldwide **epidemic***.

consequence　后果，结果；影响

*The **consequences** could be serious.*

etiology　病因学

*The most common **etiology** is trauma.*

socioeconomic　社会经济学的

*There is a known **socioeconomic** skew in prevalence and outcomes of cardiovascular disease.*

prevalence　流行

*HIV's **prevalence** is dropping in southern India.*

cervical　子宫颈的

*The **cervical** smear test is a lifesaver.*

carcinogen　致癌物质

*A **carcinogen** that can irritate your throat, eyes, and nose.*

mortality　死亡率

*Premature birth is the main cause of perinatal **mortality***.

sedentary　久坐的；静坐的

*Obesity and a **sedentary** lifestyle have been linked with an increased risk of heart disease.*

premature　过早的，提早的

*The baby was two weeks **premature***.

saturated fat　饱和脂肪

***Saturated fat** tends to raise LDL levels.*

incidence　发生率

*The **incidence** of breast cancer increases with age.*

prioritiy　优先处理的事

*It did not figure high on her list of **priorities***.

detection　察觉，发现

*Early **detection** of cancers is vitally important.*

screening　筛选；放映

*The **screening** tests have so far been fraught with difficulties.*

prognosis　预后；预知

*The **prognosis** of PTSD differs from individual to individual.*

tertiary 第三的, 第三位的, 第三级的

*Jobs are mainly created by the **tertiary** industry.*

Language Point

chronic respiratory disease 慢性呼吸道疾病

Chronic respiratory disease are chronic diseases of the airways and other structures of the lung. Some of the most common are asthma, chronic obstructive pulmonary disease, respiratory allergies, occupational lung diseases and pulmonary hypertension.

*Among men, exposure to this neglected risk factor nearly doubles the risk of **chronic respiratory disease.***

trans-fatty acids 反式脂肪酸

Trans-fatty acids are manufactured fats created during a process called hydrogenation, which is aimed at stabilizing polyunsaturated oils to prevent them from becoming rancid and to keep them solid at room temperature.

*Ordering a Diet Coke with that burger and fries might ease the guilt a little, but there are still all those **trans-fatty acids** to worry about.*

disability-adjusted life years (DALYs) 伤残调整生命年

The disability-adjusted life year (DALY) is a measure of overall disease burden, expressed as the number of years lost due to ill-health, disability, or early death.

*Methods **disability-adjusted life years (DALY)** is used as the indicator.*

survival time 生存时间

It is the percentage of people in a study or treatment group still alive for a given period after diagnosis.

*The median **survival time** was 4.0 years (1.5-8.5 years).*

life expectancy 预期寿命

Life expectancy is a statistical measure of the average time an organism is expected to live, based on the year of its birth, its current age, and other demographic factors including sex.

*Metal stent placement is only indicated for patients who are intolerant of operation, or whose **life expectancy** is less than two years.*

EXERCISES

Task 1: Vocabulary Application
Fill in the blanks with the words given below. Change the form where necessary.

trans-fatty acids; preventive; prevalence; mortality; carcinogen; genetic; insidious; diabetes; prognosis; sedentary

1. Is it possible to manage an HIV epidemic so that _____ stay low for long periods?

2. Researchers then estimated _____ intake based on overall meat consumption and doneness preferences.

3. Her cancer was discovered early and her _____ is excellent.

4. The kind of fat you should avoid is _____ .

5. He said that he would like to see data on _____ for the drug.

6. Wadsworth obtained a noni (诺丽果) sample and tested its juice on a friend who had _____ .

7. On the contrary, _____ lifestyle has been demonstrated to be a risk of diabetes and rectal cancer.

8. Chronic diseases do not occur at random and usually have causal risk and _____ factors that can be found.

9. NCDs are the results of a combination of _____ , physiological, environmental, and behavioral factors and usually characterized by _____ onset and long duration.

Task 2: Writing

One of the most important ways of reducing deaths from noncommunicable diseases (NCDs) is to control an unhealthy lifestyle. For this part, you are allowed to write a composition to express your views on how to perform interventions to support behavioral self-management. You should write at least 150 words but no more than 300 words.

Flexible and stretchable wearable sensors play an important role in endowing chronic disease care systems with the capability of long-term and real-time tracking of biomedical signals. For this part, you are allowed to write a composition to express your views on the applications of wearable sensors in chronic disease care. You should write at least 150 words but no more than 300 words.

Task 3: Oral Presentation

Lifestyle medicine presents a new and challenging approach to addressing the prevention and treatment of noncommunicable diseases. The Chronic Care Model is a reasonable system of delivery to consider for lifestyle medicine, which is composed of six components that are designed to affect functional and clinical outcomes associated with chronic disease management: healthcare organization, community resources, self-management support, delivery system design, decision support and clinical information systems. Please talk about your views on lifestyle medicine.

READING B

PREVIEW

*Stroke is the leading cause of death and long-term disability in China, which causes severe economic and social burdens. Stroke is an acute neurological deficit caused by an abnormality in the cerebral blood vessels, including arterial occlusion, **stenosis** or vascular* *rupture. **Ischemic stroke** and **intracerebral hemorrhage** are the two main types of stroke. Previous epidemiological studies have found a strong association between stroke and some potentially modifiable risk factors, suggesting that stroke could be prevented and the primary stroke prevention is a fundamental measure to reduce the risk of stroke. In addition, timely and effective treatment of stroke can prevent long-term disability and prolong lifespan. Thus, it is of great significance to conduct stroke prevention, standardize stroke diagnosis procedures and improve treatment efficacy to reduce the risk of stroke in China.*

Questions for Discussion

Q1: Talk about the understanding of stroke from clinical and epidemiological aspects.

Q2: How to make efforts to promote the prevention and treatment of stroke in China?

Text B

Brief Introduction of Stroke in China

Stroke is an important cardiovascular disease that has become one of the major global public health problems. In China, stroke remains the leading cause of death and long-term disability, and contributes to a heavy economic burden. Data from the Global Burden of Disease (GBD) Study 2016 indicated that the estimated global lifetime risk of stroke from the age of 25 years onward was 24.9% (95% uncertainty interval, 23.5% to 26.2%), while China had the highest estimated risk of up to 39.3%. With the accelerated aging and urbanization of society, as well as widespread exposure to unhealthy lifestyles and cardiovascular risk factors, the incidence and prevalence of stroke have continued to rise over the past 30 years in China. The National Epidemiological Survey of Stroke in China (NESS-China) involved 480,687 adults aged ≥20 years from 31 provinces between 2012 and 2013, reporting an age-standardized stroke prevalence of 1,115 cases per 100,000 people, an annual age-standardized incidence of 247 cases per 100,000 people, and a mortality rate of 115 cases per 100,000 people, respectively. These data suggest that there are 11.1 million living stroke survivors, 2.4 million new strokes, and 1.1 million stroke-related deaths each year. Moreover, stroke is characterized by high recurrence rates and combined cardiovascular events. Stroke places a heavy and enormous burden on the healthcare system in China. Over the past decades, Chinese experts have established the prevention and control concepts for stroke and carried out related work, and the government has taken several important steps to address stroke prevention and treatment.

Subtypes and Diagnosis

Stroke is an acute neurological deficit caused by an abnormality in the cerebral blood vessels, including arterial occlusion, stenosis, or vascular rupture. Stroke can be categorized as ischemic stroke, intracerebral hemorrhage, or **subarachnoid hemorrhage**. Ischemic stroke and intracerebral hemorrhage are the two main types of stroke. The NESS-China study indicated that ischemic stroke **accounts for** approximately 70% of all incident stroke cases and intracerebral hemorrhage accounts for 24%. Ischemic stroke is defined as an **episode** of neurological dysfunction caused by focal cerebral, spinal, or **retinal** infarction with symptoms persisting for more than 24 hours. Transient ischemic attack (TIA) is a similar event to ischemic stroke. A TIA is also a focal brain ischemia event that causes sudden, transient neurologic deficits, but is not accompanied by permanent brain infarction. The symptoms are usually transient, lasting from minutes to hours but less than 24 hours. Ischemic strokes can be further categorized according to the Trial of Org 10172 in Acute Stroke Treatment (TOAST) classification: large artery **atherosclerosis**, small-vessel occlusion, cardioembolism, stroke of other determined **etiology**, and stroke of undetermined etiology. Typical clinical features of ischemic stroke include loss of motor control and sensation in some regions of the body, visual changes and deficits, **dysarthria**, loss of consciousness, and facial droop.

Intracerebral hemorrhage is defined as rapidly developing clinical signs of neurological dysfunction attributable to a focal collection of blood within the brain **parenchyma** or **ventricular** system that is not caused by **trauma**. Although intracerebral hemorrhage accounts for 15%-30% of all strokes, it is one of the most disabling forms of stroke. It is reported that more than one third of intracerebral hemorrhage patients will not survive, and only twenty percent of patients will regain functional independence. The clinical features of intracerebral hemorrhage are similar to those of ischemic stroke. In addition, subarachnoid hemorrhage can **give rise to** the following set of signs and symptoms, including sudden onset of a severe headache, **nausea**, vomiting, **syncope**, and **photophobia**.

Risk Factors and Prevention

In a **mega**-case-control study of 13,447 patients with a first acute stroke (10,388 with ischemic stroke and 3,059 with intracerebral hemorrhage) and 13,472 controls from 32 countries, the INTERSTROKE study showed that 90.7% of the population-attributable risk of stroke is associated with ten potentially modifiable risk factors in all major regions of the world, as well as among all ethnic groups, sexes, and ages. The ten modifiable risk factors include hypertension, smoking, diabetes mellitus, physical activity, diet, psychosocial factors, abdominal obesity, alcohol, cardiac causes, and **apolipoproteins**. For the Chinese population, these ten risk factors together account for 94.3% of all strokes, 95.2% of ischemic strokes, and 90.7% of hemorrhagic strokes. These findings suggest that stroke can be prevented, and primary stroke prevention is a fundamental measure to reduce the risk of stroke.

Hypertension is the most important modifiable risk factor for all types of stroke. A nationwide survey of 451,755 residents $\geq$18 years of age from 31 provinces, autonomous regions, and municipalities in mainland of China from 2012 to 2015 reported that 23.2% ($\approx$244.5 million) of the Chinese adult population $\geq$18 years of age had hypertension, and another 41.3% ($\approx$435.3 million) had pre-hypertension according to the Chinese guideline. In addition, among individuals with hypertension, 46.9% were aware of their condition, 40.7% were taking prescribed antihypertensive medications, and only 15.3% had controlled hypertension. The NESS-China study suggested that the prevalence of hypertension in stroke survivors in China is

84%, which is higher than most other countries, and it is estimated that 73% of the stroke burden in China is attributable to hypertension. Therefore, improving blood pressure control remains a crucial strategy in China.

Data from the GBD study suggested that air pollution has emerged as a significant contributor to the global stroke burden, especially in low-income and middle-income countries. In China, almost 22% of stroke-related disability-adjusted life-years (DALYs) in 2013 were attributed to **ambient** PM 2.5 air pollution. The China Kadoorie Biobank (CKB) study reported that solid fuel use for cooking and heating was associated with higher risks of cardiovascular (including ischemic heart disease death, stroke death and other cardiovascular death) and all-cause mortality after a mean of 7.2 years of follow-up, and those switched from solid to clean fuels for cooking had a lower risk of cardiovascular mortality, and all-cause mortality in rural China. Reducing exposure to air pollution should be one of the main priorities to reduce stroke burden in China, and other low-income and middle-income countries.

Healthcare organizations and Stroke societies (such as Chinese Stroke Society, Stroke Prevention and Control Society, and the Chinese Stroke Association) have conducted varied public educational activities on stroke prevention across the country, including treating hypertension, healthy eating habits, stopping smoking, and so on. As the increasing burden of stroke in China, the primary prevention strategies still need to be improved.

Stroke Identification

Timely and effective treatment of stroke can prevent long-term disability and save lives. However, prehospital delays are common, and only a small proportion of stroke patients are aware of the initial symptoms of a stroke. Improving community awareness of initial stroke symptoms and the establishment of an alert system to **cater for** patients likely to experience stroke at home may be promising methods to help **expedite** transport to hospital. Dr. Zhao Jing from Shanghai Minhang Hospital proposed "Stroke 1-2-0" as a novel educational strategy suitable for China. The medical emergency telephone number is 120 in China, which can be adapted as a convenient **mnemonic** tool for rapid stroke recognition in Chinese. These numbers are transformed into three stroke recognition actions, where "1" represents "first, look for an uneven face", "2" represents "second, examine for arm weakness", and "0" represents "zero (absence of) clear speech". If stroke is suspected or identified through this three-step observation, the emergency number 120 must be dialed. The use of Stroke 1-2-0 as a mnemonic tool links stroke identification with the emergency service telephone number, and can be easily remembered even by those with minimal education.

Stroke Treatment

Intravenous thrombolysis (tissue-type **plasminogen** activator, tPA) has served as a primary therapy for acute ischemic stroke. While the licensed time window extends to three hours from symptom onset, recent data suggest that the trial window can be extended up to 4.5 h with overall benefit. The treatment is more effective when given early after symptom onset. After thrombolysis, 10% more patients survive and live independently. Despite its benefits, there is a risk that thrombolysis can cause bleeding. Thrombectomy is a treatment that physically removes a **clot** from the brain. It usually involves inserting a mesh device into an artery in the **groin**, moving it up to the brain, and pulling the clot out. It only works with people where the blood clot is in a large artery. Like thrombolysis, it has to be carried out within hours of a stroke starting. Only a small proportion of stroke cases are eligible for thrombectomy, but it can have a big impact on those people by reducing disability. Endovascular thrombectomy has become part of the standard treatment for patients who have acute ischemic stroke due to large-vessel occlusion in the **anterior** cerebral circulation.

Antiplatelets and **statins** are the most commonly prescribed medications in the acute phase of ischemic stroke in China. The CHANCE (Clopidogrel in High-Risk Patients with Acute Nondisabling Cerebrovascular Events) trial has recruited 5,170 patients with minor ischemic stroke or TIA from 114 centers in China, and shown that dual antiplatelet therapy with clopidogrel and aspirin was more effective for the prevention of stroke recurrence.

The management of acute intracerebral hemorrhage is challenging. Currently no medical treatments have been shown definitively to improve the outcome. The treatment principle has been focusing on stopping the bleeding, removing the clot and relieving pressure on the brain. The majority of patients suffering intracerebral hemorrhage are present with elevated BP levels in the acute phase, and about two-thirds of Chinese patients receive early antihypertensive therapy. The INTERACT2 (Intensive Blood Pressure Reduction in Acute Cerebral Hemorrhage Trial) trial, a large clinical trial assigned 2,839 intracerebral hemorrhage patients to one of two different blood pressure control strategies (systolic level < 140 mmHg within 1 hour vs. SBP < 180 mmHg). Although this trial failed to find a significant reduction in the rate of the primary outcome of death or severe disability, intensive BP lowering appeared safe, and numerous secondary outcomes appeared to be superior to the intensive strategy. Furthermore, patients with intracerebral hemorrhage are frequently recommended for surgery, such as **hemostatic** therapy and **hematoma evacuation**, but the efficacy and safety still need to be investigated.

Efforts and Future Directions

In 2009, the Ministry of Health of the People's Republic of China launched the Stroke Prevention and Treatment Project of the National Health Commission (SPTPC) to meet the challenge of stroke. SPTPC actively promotes the establishment of a stroke prevention and treatment system in China. The health committees of all provinces, autonomous regions, and municipalities directly under the central government have established stroke prevention and treatment committees/leading groups and expert groups to organize medical institutions, emergency units, disease control institutions, and primary health care units. SPTPC also carried out standardized training and promotion of prevention and treatment technology for cerebrovascular diseases, significantly improving the ability of stroke treatment. In the next step, SPTPC will continue to participate in the screening and intervention of high-risk populations of stroke, improve the construction of regional stroke prevention and control system, vigorously promote the construction of stroke center and standardize the algorithm for the stroke diagnosis, increase the treatment efficacy, consolidate quality control and standardization work, and improve the mode of mobile stroke and remote diagnosis and treatment.

In recent years, great progress has been made in the prevention and treatment of stroke in China. However, as the prevalence and incidence of stroke are still increasing, the prevention and treatment of stroke still face huge challenges, and the system needs to be further improved.

Words and Expressions

stenosis （器官）狭窄

*I developed spinal **stenosis** in my c-spine.*

rupture 使破裂

*His stomach might **rupture** from all the acid.*

episode 一段经历；发病

*Immediately following an **episode** of stroke, the innate immune system is activated.*

retinal 视网膜的

*There are potential side effects: burning and **retinal** discoloration.*

atherosclerosis 动脉粥样硬化

*Gum problems increase the risk of **atherosclerosis**.*

dysarthria 构音障碍

*The type of **dysarthria** determines the treatment.*

parenchyma 实质；软细胞组织

*The lung **parenchyma** appeared echo rich and patchy.*

ventricular 心室的；脑室的

*The patient underwent external decompression and external **ventricular** drainage.*

trauma 痛苦经历；创伤

*The patient suffered severe brain **trauma**.*

nausea 恶心

*Symptoms include **nausea** and giddiness.*

syncope 晕厥

*Most of the post-exercise syncopes were vasodepressor **syncopes**.*

photophobia 畏光

*The woman presented with **photophobia** and reduced vision.*

mega 巨大的

*He has become **mega** rich.*

apolipoprotein 载脂蛋白

*The gene transcription of **apolipoprotein** A5 is controlled by several factors.*

ambient 周围的；外界的

*The design cuts out most of the **ambient** noise.*

expedite 加快；促进

*We have developed rapid order processing to **expedite** deliveries to customers.*

mnemonic 记忆的

*Many of them use a **mnemonic** method.*

plasminogen　血纤维蛋白溶酶原

*Urokinase, a human **plasminogen** activator, is used clinically to promote the dissolution of thrombi.*

clot　凝块，血块

*They removed a **clot** from his brain.*

groin　腹股沟

*I underwent an operation on my **groin** once.*

anterior　前面的

*Cardioembolism is more frequently located in the **anterior** circulation.*

antiplatelet　抗血小板的

*There is currently no robust evidence to support the use of venous **antiplatelet** agents.*

statin　他汀类

***Statin** drugs lower cholesterol.*

hemostatic　止血的

*The speed of laser operation for cutting the department of **hemostatic** steps can be improved.*

hematoma　血肿

*That head bump is now blamed for triggering the **hematoma**.*

evacuation　清除

*Each house had a helipad for a fast **evacuation**.*

Language Point

ischemic stroke　缺血性卒中

the most common kind of stroke; caused by an interruption in the flow of blood to the brain (as from a clot blocking a blood vessel)

*Carotid artery stenosis is one of the major causes of **ischemic stroke**.*

intracerebral hemorrhage　脑出血

hemorrhage caused by non-traumatic parenchymal vascular rupture

*Clinically brain cell injury after **intracerebral hemorrhage** (ICH) always causes dysfunction or death on such patients.*

subarachnoid hemorrhage　蛛网膜下腔出血

Subarachnoid hemorrhage (SAH) is a clinical syndrome caused by rupture of pathological blood vessels at the base or surface of the brain and direct inflow of blood into the subarachnoid space, also known as primary subarachnoid hemorrhage, which is a very serious and common disease.

*Ruptured cerebral aneurysm is one of the important reasons for **subarachnoid hemorrhage**.*

accounts for　占……比例

*The brain **accounts for** merely three percent of body weight.*

give rise to　使发生，引起

*Low levels of choline in the body can **give rise to** high blood pressure.*

cater for　迎合；供应伙食；为……提供所需

*The university started some new language programs to **cater for** China's Silk Road Economic Belt.*

intravenous thrombolysis　静脉溶栓

Thrombus-dissolving drugs are used in venous tube to recanalize vascular.

*All patients were treated with **intravenous thrombolysis** therapy.*

EXERCISES

Task 1: Vocabulary Application

Fill in the blanks with the words given below. Change the form where necessary.

> **rupture; ventricular; atherosclerosis; intracerebral hemorrhage; intravenous thrombolysis; cardiovascular; photophobia; antiplatelet; ischemic stroke; retinal**

1. While guidelines acknowledge uncertainty over the safety and efficacy of intravenous alteplase in acute _____ patients with a clinical history of potential bleeding diathesis, concerns over excessive bleeding contribute to underutilization of in _____ patients with AIS.

2. Diabetes mellitus enhances coronary _____ and impairs microcirculation leading to left _____ (LV) dysfunction.

3. Achromatopsia is an early-onset, _____ dystrophy characterized by reduced visual acuity, pendular nystagmus, _____ and color blindness.

4. _____ diseases, especially acute coronary syndromes, are closely associated with atherosclerotic plaque progression and _____ .

5. At least one-third of adults in high-income countries with stroke caused by spontaneous (nontraumatic) _____ are already taking oral antithrombotic (_____ or anticoagulant) drug therapy because of their comorbidities and other risk factors for vascular disease.

Task 2: Writing

For this part, you are allowed to write a composition to express your views on how to perform primary prevention for stroke in our daily life. You should write at least 150 words but no more than 300 words.

Task 3: Oral Presentation

Observational studies have reported that elevated BP is associated with adverse short-and long-term clinical outcomes after acute ischemic stroke. However, clinical trials have generally found a neutral effect of early blood pressure decrease on clinical outcomes after acute ischemic stroke. On one hand, BP-decreasing treatment may reduce vascular damage, cerebral edema, and hemorrhagic transformation of the cerebral infarction. On the other hand, early BP reduction may also decrease cerebral perfusion of the ischemic tissue and further increase the size of the cerebral infarction. Please debate whether it is necessary to decrease BP early after stroke.

Learning Garden

The Framingham Heart Study

The Framingham Heart Study is a long-term, ongoing cardiovascular cohort study of residents of the city of Framingham, Massachusetts. The study began in 1948 with 5,209 men and women between the ages of 30 and 62 from Framingham and is now on its third generation of participants. In the past 70 years, the total number of participants in FHS has reached 15,447, and the loss to follow-up rate of the first generation of participants is less than 4%. Before the study, almost nothing was known about the epidemiology of hypertensive or arteriosclerotic cardiovascular disease. Over the years, the study has illuminated that most cardiovascular disease is caused by modifiable risk factors such as smoking, obesity, lack of physical activity, high blood pressure, and high cholesterol levels. Risk factors for other physiological conditions such as dementia have continued to be investigated.

（周涛、仲崇科）

Unit 3　Epidemiology of Infectious Diseases

READING A

PREVIEW

The epidemiology of infectious diseases is concerned with the study of the occurrence, development, and distribution of infectious diseases within a population with the ultimate goal of preventing and controlling their spread. The epidemiological process involves three essential components: the source of infection, the mode of transmission, and the susceptible population. ***Pathogens*** *such as bacteria, viruses,* ***mycoplasmas****, and* ***parasites*** *are the causative agents of infectious diseases and can be transmitted via* ***respiratory*** *transmission,* ***gastrointestinal*** *transmission, insect-borne transmission, and body fluid transmission.*

Epidemiology of infectious diseases is a practical science aimed at reducing the impact of pathogens on public health and well-being. Traditional epidemiology of infectious diseases has focused primarily on the measurement of biological, environmental, and behavioral risk factors at the individual level. However, recent research has shown that infectious diseases are not only public health problems but also social problems, such as the case of acquired ***immunodeficiency*** *syndrome (AIDS). Researchers in the field are increasingly interested in* ***elucidating*** *the social* ***context*** *of infectious disease transmission, risk factors, and health* ***inequities****.*

Text A

The Concept of Infectious Diseases, Epidemic Characteristics and Epidemic Process

The term "infectious disease" refers to a range of illnesses caused by pathogens that can be transmitted between humans, between animals, or from animals to humans. Despite the **significant** progress made in the prevention and control of infectious diseases globally, such as the **eradication** of smallpox, and the effective control of diphtheria, pertussis, tetanus, polio, and plague, the current threat of infectious diseases remains pressing. In recent years, there has been a **resurgence** of syphilis, gonorrhea, and schistosomiasis, as well as ongoing high rates of tuberculosis and viral hepatitis. Additionally, the emergence of new infectious diseases such as Ebola hemorrhagic fever, legionnaires disease, AIDS, Lyme disease, highly pathogenic avian influenza, severe acute respiratory syndrome, and COVID-19 has added to the dual threat of both old and new infectious diseases.

According to the intensity and breadth of the epidemic process, the epidemiological characteristics of infectious diseases can be classified as sporadic, epidemic, pandemic and outbreak. A sporadic refers to an incidence level of an infectious disease that is **consistent** with the general level of the calendar year, without any obvious correlations between cases in terms of time and place of onset. An epidemic is an incidence of an infectious disease in a specific area that exceeds the incidence level of the same period in the calendar year, with clear **temporal** and spatial links between cases. A pandemic is characterized by a rapid spread of an infectious disease across wide geographical areas, including across provincial, national, or even continental boundaries, and with a greater intensity than an epidemic. An **outbreak** refers to the sudden appearance of a large number of patients with similar symptoms in a short period of time in a localized area or unit, with a common source of infection or transmission route.

The occurrence of infectious diseases in a population is dependent on the convergence of three **fundamental** conditions, referred to as the three links of the epidemic process. These three links in disease occurrence include the source of infection, the method of transmission, and the presence of a susceptible population. When these three **components** coexist and interact, they can result in the outbreak of infectious diseases.

The source of infection is the body of the pathogen growth, reproduction and discharge of pathogens of people or animals, including patients with infectious diseases, carriers of pathogens and infected animals. Patients with infectious diseases are important sources of infection, such as diphtheria, tuberculosis and other respiratory infectious diseases when patients cough can **discharge** a large number of pathogens, increasing the chances of susceptible people being infected. The significance of a patient as a source of infection can be influenced by several factors, including the number of pathogens excreted, the virulence of the pathogens, and the range of activity of the patient. In the progression of an infectious disease, the patient's condition can typically be divided into three phases: the **incubation** period, the clinical symptoms period, and the recovery period, each with its own varying levels of pathogen **excretion**. In addition to infected individuals, carriers of pathogens such as bacteria, viruses, mycoplasma and spirochetes also play a role in the transmission of infectious diseases. Carriers of pathogens can be divided into three categories: latent carriers of infectious diseases, recovering carriers, and healthy carriers. Infected animals can also serve as a source of infection for certain human infectious diseases. The pathogens of some diseases are mainly transmitted among animals in nature and can be transmitted to humans under certain conditions, resulting in diseases called natural epidemic diseases or **zoonotic** diseases, such as plague, brucellosis, forest encephalitis, leptospirosis, schistosomiasis, rabies, etc.

The transmission route refers to the process by which pathogens are transmitted from an infected source to a **susceptible** host. It **encompass**es the entire journey that the pathogen undergoes in the external environment after being discharged from the infectious source and before invading a new host. The transmission route of an infectious disease can be complex and can vary based on multiple factors. Each infectious disease can be transmitted by one or more routes of transmission.

In general, transmission routes are classified into two categories: **vertical** transmission and

horizontal transmission. Vertical transmission, also known as mother-to-child transmission or perinatal transmission, refers to the transfer of pathogens from a mother to her offspring during the perinatal period. This type of transmission can be further classified into three subcategories: transplacental transmission, upstream transmission, and transmission during childbirth. Horizontal transmission, on the other hand, refers to the transmission of pathogens from one person to another. This type of transmission can occur through various routes, including airborne transmission, contact transmission, waterborne transmission, foodborne transmission, and vector-borne arthropod transmission.

Airborne transmission is a crucial mode of transmission for respiratory infectious diseases (e.g., measles, chickenpox, influenza, etc.) and includes droplets, droplet nuclei, and dust. The characteristics of airborne infectious diseases include **extensive dissemination**, facile achievement of the transmission route, and a high rate of incidence. In addition, airborne infectious diseases are seasonally distinct, commonly occurring in winter and spring; have a cyclical increase in incidence in populations without immunization and **prophylaxis**; and tend to occur in areas with crowded living and high population density.

Transmission by contact can be divided into direct contact transmission and indirect contact transmission according to whether the pathogen stays in the external environment before invading the susceptible host organism after leaving the infectious source.

Direct contact transmission occurs when the pathogen is transmitted directly from the source of infection to the susceptible host without the involvement of external factors, such as in the case of rabies or sexually transmitted diseases, etc. On the other hand, indirect contact transmission takes place as a result of contact with objects **contaminated** with pathogens, which is often the case in many intestinal, respiratory, and skin infectious diseases. This mode of transmission is usually caused by contact with everyday objects contaminated with pathogens.

Waterborne transmission is the main route of transmission for many **intestinal** infectious diseases (such as cholera, typhoid, dysentery, hepatitis A, etc.) and certain parasitic diseases (such as schistosomiasis, leptospirosis, etc.). Waterborne infectious diseases have two transmission routes, namely drinking water contaminated with pathogens and contact with water contaminated with pathogens. Waterborne diseases are often epidemic outbreaks, and their epidemiological characteristics are: case distribution and water supply range consistent with a history of drinking the same water source or contact with infected water; except for nursing infants, the onset of disease without age and gender differences, more cases of drinking raw water; in the case of water sources are often contaminated, cases often continue to appear, strengthen the treatment of infected water and personal protection, can control the occurrence of cases; acute onset is often seasonal, regional and occupational, with patients mostly seen in water network areas, during the rainy season and after disasters, and the onset is mostly seen in occupational groups exposed to infected water. Transmission through contact with pathogen-infected water is usually due to the invasion of pathogens (e.g., schistosomes and **leptospira**) through the skin and mucous membranes when people come into contact with water containing specific pathogens.

Foodborne transmission is a key mode of transmission for a range of intestinal infectious diseases, including typhoid fever and bacterial dysentery, as well as certain parasitic diseases, such as pig tapeworm. The hallmark features of foodborne infectious diseases are: the presence of a history of consuming contaminated food, with only those who consume the contaminated food developing the disease; a short incubation period, which is often seen during the summer and fall; outbreaks that can occur among diners and can be effectively curtailed when the supply of contaminated food is discontinued; moreover, when the food is repeatedly contaminated, persistent outbreaks and epidemics can occur.

Vector-borne arthropod transmission, also known as insect-borne transmission, refers to infectious diseases that are transmitted through the mechanical carrying or biting of blood by vector arthropods, such as mosquitoes, flies, fleas, cicadas, mites, and cockroaches. This mode of transmission is a major route of transmission for a range of intestinal infectious diseases, zoonotic diseases, and parasitic diseases. Vector-borne transmission can be divided into two categories: biological and mechanical.

Biological transmission, also known as blood-sucking transmission, occurs when the pathogen enters the arthropod host, where it develops and reproduces, before being transmitted to susceptible individuals. Diseases transmitted through this mode include plague, epidemic B encephalitis, forest encephalitis, malaria, typhus, and filariasis. Mechanical transmission means that some arthropods (such as flies and cockroaches) can carry pathogens, but the pathogens cannot develop and reproduce in their bodies, and only contaminate food or eating utensils through contact, regurgitation or discharge of pathogens with feces when foraging, and people are infected by ingesting contaminated food or using contaminated eating utensils, such as typhoid fever and dysentery.

The term "susceptible individuals" refers to those individuals who lack immunity to a specific pathogen and are thus at risk of infection. For example, individuals who have not had measles or received measles **vaccination** are considered susceptible to the disease. The level of susceptibility in a population is referred to as "population susceptibility". It's determined by the proportion of the population that lacks immunity to the pathogen. A high level of herd immunity within a population reduces the level of population susceptibility, while a low level of herd immunity increases it. The susceptibility level of a population can be evaluated by analyzing past disease prevalence, vaccination status, and antibody level test results of the population for the specific disease in question.

Words and Expressions

pathogen　病原体
Pathogens are the source of many infectious diseases.
mycoplasma　支原体；霉形体
Mycoplasma pneumonia in children accounts for 10% to 40% of community-acquired pneumonia in children.
parasite　寄生生物；寄生虫；寄生植物；依赖他人过活者

*Freshwater fish must be cooked to prevent **parasites**.*

respiratory　呼吸的

***Respiratory** transmitted diseases are most likely to appear in winter and spring.*

gastrointestinal　胃肠的

*The most common **gastrointestinal** symptom of chronic gastritis is indigestion.*

immunodeficiency　免疫缺陷

*Opportunistic infections are often seen in patients with **immunodeficiency**.*

elucidate　阐明；解释；说明

*Please **elucidate** the reasons for your ridiculous decision.*

context　上下文；语境；（事情发生的）背景，环境，来龙去脉

*The cultural **context** of smoking control is a very important area of research.*

inequity　不公正的事；不公正；不公平

*Different regional levels of economic development bring health **inequity**.*

significant　重要的，有重大意义的；显著的，值得注意的

*Environmental pollution remains a **significant** global problem.*

eradication　根除，消（扑）灭

*The **eradication** of infectious diseases is not an easy task.*

resurgence　复苏；复兴；重新抬头

*The **resurgence** of sexually transmitted diseases poses a serious public health challenge.*

consistent　一致的；始终如一的；连续的；持续的

*A person's behavior is basically **consistent** with his principles.*

temporal　时间的；世俗的；世间的；现世的

*The epidemic of infectious disease should be analyzed from different **temporal** perspectives.*

outbreak　（暴力、疾病等坏事的）暴发，突然发生

*Spoiled food led to this **outbreak** of food poisoning.*

fundamental　十分重大的；根本的；基础的；基本的

*The current **fundamental** route of HIV transmission is unprotected sexual contact.*

components　组成部分；成分；部件

*The precise relationship of cardiac **components** is a guarantee of cardiac function.*

discharge　释放；排出；履行；流出

*The sneeze of a person with a respiratory infection can **discharge** huge amounts of pathogens.*

incubation　孵（卵）；孵化；（传染病的）潜伏期；（细菌等的）繁殖

*The illness has an **incubation** period of up to 7 days.*

excretion　排泄，排泄物；分泌，分泌物

*Urine is an important **excretion** that monitors the health of the body.*

zoonotic　动物传染病的；人畜共患病的

*Rabies is a **zoonotic** disease that is transmitted between animals and humans.*

susceptible　易受影响；敏感；过敏；好动感情的；善感的

*Weak people are more **susceptible** to contract respiratory infections.*

encompass　包含，包括，涉及（大量事物）；包围；围绕；围住

*The transmissions of HIV **encompass** sexual, blood and mother-to-child transmission.*

vertical　竖的；垂直的；直立的；纵向的

*Mother-to-child transmission of syphilis is a **vertical** transmission.*

horizontal　水平的；与地面平行的；横的

*Please place the armrests in a **horizontal** position to ensure safety when landing the aircraft.*

extensive　广阔的；广大的；大量的；广泛的；广博的

*There are **extensive** galaxies and stars in the universe.*

dissemination　传播；散播；

*Most science materials written for public **dissemination** should be easy to understand.*

prophylaxis　（疾病）预防

*Pre-exposure **prophylaxis** can reduce HIV transmission in high-risk populations.*

contaminated　污染；弄脏；玷污，毒害，腐蚀

*Drinking water near this gold mine has been **contaminated** with mercury.*

intestinal　肠道的；肠的

Parasites in the **intestinal** tract can cause serious health problems.

leptospira　钩端螺旋体；细螺旋体

Leptospirosis is a zoonotic disease caused by pathogenic species of **leptospira**.

vaccination　接种疫苗；注射疫苗；种痘

Vaccination is very effective as a method of preventing smallpox.

Language Points

acquired immunodeficiency syndrome　获得性免疫缺陷综合征

Acquired immunodeficiency syndrome is a serious infection disease in which the body's immune system is destroyed by human immunodeficiency virus, resulting in a combination of symptoms such as opportunistic infections and tumors that can eventually lead to death.

Acquired immunodeficiency syndrome was first seen in gay men in the United States, and the leading cause of death is Pneumocystis carinii pneumonia or Kaposi sarcoma.

incubation period　潜伏期

Incubation period is the period between infection and the appearance of symptoms of the disease.

*There is usually an **incubation period** of 1-10 years after HIV infection, and infected people often have no obvious symptoms.*

vertical transmission　垂直传播

Vertical transmission is a transmission route of an agent from an individual to its offspring, that is, from one generation to the next.

*There are currently technologies that can be applied to stop the **vertical transmission** of HIV and prevent infection in infants.*

intestinal infectious diseases 肠道传染病

Infectious diseases in which the pathogen invades the intestine through the mouth and can excrete pathogens from the feces, including cholera, bacterial dysentery, typhoid, paratyphoid, viral hepatitis, etc.

Intestinal infectious diseases are most prevalent in young children aged 1-4 years.

population susceptibility 人群易感性

Population susceptibility is the degree of susceptibility to an infectious disease in a population. A person who lacks specific immunity to an infectious disease and is susceptible to the disease is called a susceptible person to that infectious disease.

The high *population susceptibility* to a novel virus requires us to keep a close eye on its epidemiological situation.

EXERCISES

Task 1: Vocabulary Application

Fill in the blanks with the words given below. Change the form where necessary.

> **Candidate words:**
> consistent; inequity; contaminated; extensive; parasites; vaccination; zoonotic; susceptible; vertical; resurgence

1. Health _____ among immigration is a common problem globally, especially in the distribution of health resources.

2. Each year, roughly one in six people in this poor area of the African country gets sick from eating _____ food.

3. The _____ axis of the graph generally has a clear scale, indicating the frequency.

4. The medical community needs to be alerted to the _____ of diseases such as tuberculosis.

5. It is unreasonable that what you say is not _____ with what you do.

6. He writes very good essays, mainly because he has an _____ vocabulary.

7. There are _____ in raw meat and fish as well as raw vegetables.

8. Young people are perhaps most _____ by advertisements and buy useless items.

9. Control of _____ diseases is one of the important tasks in the field of public health.

10. People's willingness of _____ is often related to their level of health awareness and perceived threat of disease.

Task 2: Writing

For this part, you are allowed 30 minutes to write a composition on the topic: HIV/AIDS. You should write at least 120 words, and base your composition on the outline below:

1) What is HIV/AIDS?

2) How is HIV transmitted in the population?

3) What are the prevention and control strategies for HIV/AIDS?

Task 3: Oral Presentation

From your point of view, explain the necessity and urgency of HIV/AIDS prevention among the youth population.

READING B

PREVIEW

Viral hepatitis is a group of infectious liver diseases caused by five different hepatitis viruses and has liver inflammation as the major damage. These hepatitis viruses (HAV–HEV) belong to five different virus families and they are genomically distinct with different replication strategies. They also have different clinical features and outcomes. hepatitis A virus (HAV) and hepatitis E virus (HEV) infections are transient, and hepatitis B virus (HBV) and hepatitis C virus (HCV) and hepatitis D virus (HDV) infections can be transient or chronic. Viral hepatitis occurs worldwide and it is a significant public health problem in many countries, resulting in considerable morbidity and mortality. Its epidemiological features in China are as follows: high prevalence, high infectivity, multiple routes of transmission and a great health burden. HBV is the most prevalent of the three viruses known to cause chronic hepatitis, and the other two are HCV and HDV. HBV and related liver cirrhosis and hepatocellular carcinoma cause approximately 300,000 deaths annually in China. More efforts are needed to improve and develop strategies for the control of HBV infection in China.

Questions for Discussion

Q1: Which group is at a higher risk of hepatitis B?

Q2: What do you think is the reason for the high prevalence of hepatitis B in China?

Text B

The Prevalence and Control of HBV in China

For centuries, hepatitis was a mystery and understanding came in waves until its origin was finally unraveled. The first description was found in Sumer (3rd millennium B.C.) with the first description of **jaundice** on clay tablets that were the first handbook of medicine. However, the individualization of several types of hepatitis only emerged after World War II. Based on a major outbreak of hepatitis in the US Navy, Mac Callum suggested the first historical distinction between two forms of hepatitis in 1947: epidemic hepatitis with a short incubation and **serum** hepatitis with a long incubation (100-day fever). And up to now, hepatitis B virus (HBV) infection has been the most common chronic **viral** infection and a major public health problem in the world. Hepatitis C virus (HCV) and HBV are the leading causes of liver cancer and overall mortality globally, surpassing **malaria** and **tuberculosis**. An updated estimate indicated that the total global HBV infection prevalence increased to 3.9%, corresponding to 292 million people globally, suggesting that the presence of HBV was not decreasing. In addition, it was found that only 4.8 million (5%) of those eligible for treatment had actually been treated. Approximately three-quarters of individuals with chronic HBV worldwide are found in the Asia-Pacific region, particularly in the Western Pacific region, which is comprised of 37 countries including China, Japan, Republic of Korea, Philippines, and Vietnam.

The **infectious** source of hepatitis B is mainly people with HBV in their bodies, including patients with **acute** and **chronic** hepatitis B and HBV **carriers**. Among them, the most infectious are the **latent** late stage and early stage of acute hepatitis B. And chronic patients and viral carriers are the most important sources of infection, and their infectivity is directly **proportional** to viral load and HBV DNA content in body fluid. Most people do not experience any symptoms when newly infected and have no evidence of liver disease or injury. However, some people have acute illness that last several weeks with symptoms, including yellowing of the skin and eyes (jaundice), dark urine, extreme **fatigue**, loss of appetite, **nausea**, **vomiting**, and **abdominal** pain. **Malaise** and **anorexia** might precede jaundice by 1-2 weeks. Jaundice is not common in young children with acute HBV infection. It is more common in adults and older children. In the process of HBV infection, people with acute hepatitis can develop acute liver failure which can lead to death. **Extrahepatic** manifestations of disease (e.g., skin **rash**, **arthralgias**, and **arthritis**) also might occur. Among the long-term **complication**s of HBV infections, a subset of persons develops advanced liver diseases such as cirrhosis and hepatocellular carcinoma, which cause high **morbidity** and **mortality**.

HBV is **transmitted** through contact with infected blood or body **secretions**. Three major modes of transmission prevail. In areas of high endemicity, HBV is transmitted mostly **perinatally** from infected mothers to **neonates**. In low-endemic areas, sexual transmission is predominant. The risk of infection is higher in people with a high number of sexual partners, men who have sex with men, and people with a history of other sexually transmitted infections. The third major source of infection is unsafe injections, blood **transfusions**, or **dialysis**. Although screening of blood products has substantially reduced transfusion-associated HBV infection, infection in this manner is still frequent in developing countries. In addition, with the global opioid crisis, **intravenous** drug use has again become a more common mode of transmission. Other possible sources of HBV include **nosocomial** infection through contaminated medical, surgical, or dental instruments; needle-stick injuries; and organs donated by HBV surface antigen (HBsAg)-positive or HBV-DNA-positive donors. Household or intimate non-sexual contact and living in crowded conditions are also possible risks. HBV infection can be prevented by avoiding transmission from infected people and by inducing immunity in unexposed people. The implementation of universal HBV vaccination in infants has resulted in a sharp fall in prevalence in many parts of the world. The WHO recommends the use of monovalent HBV vaccination within 24 hours of birth, followed by completion of the HBV **vaccine** series within 6 to 12 months as the most cost-effective strategy for the prevention and control of hepatitis B. This strategy provides the earliest possible protection to future birth cohorts and reduces the pool of chronic carriers in the population. Currently, most countries have implemented universal neonatal HBV vaccination programs, which are inexpensive, and which may **eradicate** HBV infection within the next century.

Hepatitis B is infectious and universally susceptible, so all people may be infected by HBV. The hepatitis B susceptible population was negative for HBsAg, HBV core antibody, and HBV surface antibody. And high-risk groups for HBV infection include intravenous drug users, infants born to infected mothers, males who have sexual intercourse with other males, **hemodialysis** patients (and workers), healthcare workers, household contacts of patients known with chronic HBV infection. After acute HBV infection, significantly, infants are more likely to develop chronic HBV infection. Studies have shown that hepatitis B infection acquired in adulthood leads to chronic hepatitis in less than 5% of cases, whereas infection in infancy and early childhood leads to chronic hepatitis in about 95% of cases. Despite the use of passive-active **immunoprophylaxis** with HBV **immunoglobulin** and HBV vaccine, babies born to mothers with high HBV DNA **titers** ($>10^7$ copies per mL) still carry a substantial risk of infection. The risk of perinatal transmission might be further reduced by giving **antiviral** therapy to mothers with high **viremia** during the third trimester of pregnancy. Screening of high-risk groups for HBsAg and implementation of universal **precautions** resulted in a substantial reduction in transmission in healthcare settings. In particular, screening blood donors, increasing the detection of HBV DNA during screening processes will further reduce the incidence rate of transfusion-associated disease.

The prevalence of chronic HBV infection is higher in China, with nearly 70 million HBV carriers in 2020, affecting 4.96% of China's population of 1.41 billion people. Historically, HBV carriers have experienced discrimination when applying for jobs or educational opportunities. Many employers and universities have refused to accept anyone with a positive HBV test, and some kindergartens have refused to admit children who are carriers. Some **pharmaceutical** companies have exploited the prevalence of hepatitis B to peddle alleged cures and **remedies**. Their advertisements exaggerated the contagious nature of the disease and claimed that a large proportion of HBV carriers later have cirrhosis or hepatocellular carcinoma. As a result, misleading information has become widespread throughout China. However, the situation has improved significantly since the Chinese government has taken steps to eradicate discrimination against HBV carriers in employment and education since 2007 and additional regulations in February 2010. However, HBV-related discrimination still exists in our daily life. The most effective way to eliminate HBV-related discrimination is to fundamentally inhibit the occurrence of hepatitis B. The HBV vaccination is the most cost-effective way to prevent HBV infection. The Chinese government has listed the application of the HBV vaccine as a priority of public health works. It has made substantial progress in controlling HBV infections over the past few decades. Since 1992, when the Chinese government prioritized implementing HBV vaccinations for newborns, China began to see a more significant reduction in HBV infections. Based on the surveys conducted by China CDC since the 1990s, the seroprevalence of HBsAg among children$<$15 years old has declined from 10.5% in 1992 to 0.8% in 2014 and reached 0.3%

among children under age 5 in 2014. The overall seroprevalence of anti-HCV antibodies fell from 3.2% in 1996 to 0.43% in 2006. Meanwhile, the vaccination rate of the hepatitis B vaccine is increasing. According to the hepatitis B serological epidemiology data in 2006 and 2014, the timely vaccination rate of the first dose Hepatitis B vaccine in China increased from 22% in 1992 to 91% in 2013. The three-dose rate increased from 30% in 1992 to 95% in 2013. Data from the National Vaccination Information System of the national vaccination programmer show that between 2015 and 2018, the reported on-time vaccination rate and complete vaccination rate for the first dose of HBV in newborns remained above 90% and 95%, respectively. China is expected to achieve the prevention and control target of HBsAg positive rate <0.1% in children under five years old by 2030. While strengthening the routine **immunization** of newborns against HBV, the Chinese government has also begun to focus on strengthening adult HBV immunization programs. They were developing large-scale dissemination of knowledge about true and false HBV transmission routes and paying more attention to the critical discriminating populations. The World Health Organization called for the global elimination of viral hepatitis by 2030, and China will be a significant contributor to the global elimination of hepatitis B by 2030.

HBV infection is a major public health problem worldwide. China has the world's largest burden of HBV infection and will be a major contributor towards the global elimination of hepatitis B disease by 2030. The Chinese government should further raise the awareness and knowledge of HBV testing and treatment among the public and improve reimbursement policies or set up a special government fund to improve the affordability of care and hence patient **compliance**. In conclusion, China has made good progress in reducing HBV incidence in the past three decades. However, the country still faces challenges to achieve its target of a 65% reduction in HBV mortality by 2030. To eliminate the gap in mortality, we suggest that priority should be given to achieving the service coverage targets of diagnosis and treatment. Meanwhile, it is necessary to **integrate** existing programs and resources to establish a system that covers prevention, screening, diagnosis, and treatment of HBV infection across the life cycle. These measures will help us to make continuous progress toward the goal of eliminating hepatitis B by 2030 in China.

Words and Expressions

jaundice 黄疸
*She presented with a clinical picture of fever and **jaundice**.*
serum 血清
*The red blood cells have not separated from the **serum**.*
viral 病毒的；病毒性的；病毒引起的
*A **viral** illness left her barely able to walk.*
malaria 疟疾
***Malaria** is endemic in many hot countries.*

tuberculosis   结核病

*As late as the 1950s, **tuberculosis** was still a fatal illness.*

carrier   带菌者, 病原携带者(自身不受感染而传播疾病的人或动物)

*The badger is a **carrier** of TB.*

latent   潜在的; 潜伏的

*An important use of such data is to find indicators for **latent** diseases early on.*

proportional   成比例的; 相称的

*The size of the nebula at this stage is inversely **proportional** to its mass.*

fatigue   疲乏, 厌倦

*She continued to have severe stomach cramps, aches, **fatigue**, and depression.*

nausea   恶心; 反胃

*A wave of **nausea** swept over her.*

vomit   呕吐

*Nausea and **vomiting** are common symptoms.*

abdominal   腹部的

*She was advised to have an **abdominal** X-ray.*

malaise   乏力; 不适

*He complained of depression, headaches and **malaise**.*

anorexia   厌食; 食欲缺乏; 食欲缺乏

*People who have **anorexia** or bulimia are at risk of bone loss.*

extrahepatic   (发生或位于)肝外的

*Most often this is due to **extrahepatic** biliary tract obstruction.*

rash   皮疹; 疹

*Her face broke out in a **rash**.*

arthralgia   (外科)关节痛

***Arthralgia** and bone pain may occur.*

arthritis   (外科)关节炎

*His hands were gnarled with **arthritis**.*

complication   并发症

*Blindness is a common **complication** of diabetes.*

morbidity   发病率

*Researchers found that polyphenols in apple can lower the **morbidity** of colorectal cancer.*

transmit   传播; 传染; 传送; 输送; 发射; 播送; 传(热、声等); 透(光等); 使通过

*All the evidence argued against the theory that the disease was **transmitted** by water.*

secretion   人体分泌物; 分泌

*The **secretion** of sweat from our sweat glands helps regulate body temperature during physical activity.*

perinatal   临产的; 围生期的

*The **perinatal** mortality was as high as 51%.*

neonate   (尤指刚出生一周至四周的)新生儿

*Hypertension in **neonates** is increasingly recognized.*

transfusion （临床）输血

*He contracted AIDS from a blood **transfusion**.*

dialysis 渗析；透析（尤指将废物从肾病患者的血液中分离出来）

*I was on **dialysis** for seven years before my first transplant.*

intravenous 静脉内的

*The patient is sedated with **intravenous** use of sedative drugs.*

nosocomial 医院的；来自医院等卫生单位的（疾病或病原）

*Hospitals world-wide battle **nosocomial** infections on a daily basis.*

vaccine 疫苗

*Researchers around the world are collaborating to develop a new **vaccine**.*

eradicate 根除；消灭；杜绝

*Surely, we will aim to finally **eradicate** disease and poverty.*

hemodialysis （临床）血液透析；血液渗析

*The plasma is filtered using standard **hemodialysis** equipment.*

immunoprophylaxis 免疫预防，接种免疫；（免疫）免疫预防法

*To explore the risk of HBV transmission in breast-fed infants of chronic HBV carries after combination **immunoprophylaxis**.*

immunoglobulin （免疫）（生化）免疫球蛋白

*These abnormal LPL cells produce large amounts of the protein **immunoglobulin** and macroglobulin.*

titer 滴定量；滴度

*The immunity serum **titer** was mensured by the routine ELISA.*

antiviral 抗病毒的；抗滤过性病原体的

***Antiviral** therapy has little beneficial effects.*

viremia （医）病毒血症

*High-dose interferon can inhibit **viremia**, make an illness see better.*

precaution 预防措施，防备；避孕措施

*Asian countries should take necessary **precaution**.*

pharmaceutical 制药的

*These discoveries have stimulated the interest of academia and the **pharmaceutical** industry.*

remedy 解决方法；治疗（法）；药品

*Pickle juice has long been touted as a fix for cramping muscles, and now a recent study lends even more credibility to this home **remedy**.*

immunization 免疫

*The department is reviewing its policy with regard to **immunization**.*

compliance 用药依从性；依从性

*To investigate that the intervention would increase self-efficacy and **compliance** of self-care in patients with hypertension.*

integrate　合并；整合

*The strategy is to **integrate** the development of these cities for a better economic structure.*

Language Points

acute liver failure　急性肝功能衰竭

Acute liver failure (ALF) refers to a clinical syndrome group caused by massive necrosis of liver cells or severe damage of liver function in a short period of time due to the action of various pathogenic factors on the body.

***Acute liver failure** leads to hepatic encephalopathy.*

cirrhosis　肝硬化

A chronic disease interfering with the normal functioning of the liver; the major cause is chronic alcoholism.

*The degree of liver inflammation can range from mild to deadly, and **cirrhosis** of the liver can result.*

intravenous drug　静脉注射药物

Intravenous drug refers to a drug that is administered directly into a person's veins, typically through an injection. This method allows the drug to quickly enter the bloodstream, providing a rapid and efficient way to deliver medication or treatment.

*The patient's condition was critical, so the doctor decided to administer the medication as an **intravenous drug** to ensure it took effect quickly.*

HBsAg（Hepatitis B surface antigen）　乙型肝炎病毒表面抗原

HBsAg is the surface antigen of the hepatitis B virus. Its presence in blood indicates current hepatitis B infection.

*His blood test came back positive for **HBsAg**, indicating a current hepatitis B infection.*

perinatal transmission　围生期传播

A vertically transmitted infection is an infection caused by bacteria, viruses, or in rare cases, parasites transmitted directly from the mother to an embryo, fetus, or baby during pregnancy or childbirth. It can occur when the mother gets an infection as an intercurrent disease in pregnancy. Nutritional deficiencies may exacerbate the risks of perinatal infection.

*Lamivudine therapy might not prevent **perinatal transmission** of HBV infection in every newborn.*

seroprevalence　血清阳性率

Seroprevalence is the number of persons in a population who test positive for a specific disease based on serology (blood serum) specimens; often presented as a percent of the total specimens tested or as a proportion per 100,000 persons tested.

***Seroprevalence** presents a strong spatial correlation in lake region with certain yearly variability, but such spatial correlation is weak in mountainous region.*

EXERCISES

Task 1: Vocabulary Application

Fill in the blanks with the words given below. Change the form where necessary.

> infectious; transmit; eradicate; immunization; integrate; proportional; compliance; morbidity; precaution; remedy

1. People ill with TB bacteria in their lungs can _____ others when they cough.

2. They promote social _____ and assimilation of minority ethnic groups into the culture.

3. Rock samples taken from the remains of an asteroid about twice the size of the 6-nuke-wide asteroid that _____ the dinosaurs have been dated to be 3.47 billion years old.

4. Even though scientists play a part in _____ information to journalists and ultimately the public, too often the blame for ineffective communication is placed on the side of the journalists.

5. The monkeys used in those experiments had previously been _____ with a vaccine made from killed infected cells.

6. Although a small proportion of the total population, this perhaps had a massive local impact when a large _____ of the young men were removed from an area.

7. Vaccination remains important as a means of reducing the _____ and mortality caused by influenza viruses.

8. It is important to drive in _____ with the traffic laws, which is a responsible behavior for life.

9. Before the storm reaches them, they have been enabled to take _____ measures for its reception.

10. The forest is playing vital role in maintaining natural ecological balance, improving ecological environment, preventing and _____ pollution etc.

Task 2: Writing

For this part, you are allowed 30 minutes to write a composition on the topic: hepatitis B. You should write at least 120 words, and base your composition on the outline below:

1) What is hepatitis B?

2) What are the main routes of transmission of hepatitis B?

3) What measures have been taken to control hepatitis B in China?

Task 3: Oral Presentation

Hepatitis B virus (HBV) infection is a major global public health problem and nearly 2.57 billion people worldwide are estimated to be infected with HBV. In your opinion, what is the key to controlling its epidemics?

Learning Garden

What you need to know about HIV testing

A strong global commitment to end AIDS has driven tremendous progress in countries to prevent and control the disease. In 2019, about 81% of people living with HIV globally knew their viral status, and the remaining 19% (about 7.1 million people) still needed access to HIV testing services. At the end of 2019, 67% of people infected globally had access to antiretroviral treatment, and 12.6 million more were not receiving treatment. However, the number of new HIV infections is not declining fast enough, and too many people are still dying from AIDS-related illnesses despite high-quality and effective treatment. And with about 40 million men, women and children infected with HIV worldwide, more people are living with HIV than ever before. One in four people don't even know they are infected with the virus. People living with HIV should not die from AIDS, and people who are HIV negative should be supported with the HIV prevention knowledge and tools they need to stay negative.

Testing is the only way to determine if you have HIV. If you think you may be at risk for HIV, it is important to find out your HIV status and, if you test positive, to start treatment as soon as possible. The sooner you start treatment, the healthier you will be and the less likely you are to spread the virus. If you are pregnant or considering having a child, it is important to get tested for HIV so you know if you need to take antiretroviral drugs to prevent transmitting the virus to your child and, importantly, to keep yourself healthy in the long term by staying on ongoing antiretroviral treatment. People who test negative for HIV should connect with HIV prevention services and continue to protect themselves from HIV.

（蔡泳、褚敏捷）

Unit 4　Occupational and Environmental Hygiene

READING A

PREVIEW

Occupational health was also called industrial hygiene in the early days. Its main task is to provide workers with a safe and healthy workplace that meets sanitary standards. The focus of its work is to predict, identify, evaluate, and control occupational hazard in the workplace, that is, to protect the health of workers by improving the working environment, controlling and preventing harmful factors that may cause injury or disease or affect workers' health at work, and reducing and controlling occupational health risks. The main work of occupational health is primary prevention, including assessing possible occupational hazards and taking prevention and control measures beforehand; identifying the types of potential hazards in the workplace; assessing the degree of hazards in the workplace; and controlling the occurrence of occupational hazards. Occupational health workers need to identify, evaluate, and control occupational hazards to improve working conditions, prevent occupational diseases, and increase work efficiency, and further to predict occupational health hazards and take necessary precautionary measures to prevent occupational injuries and protect workers' health, thereby aiming to achieve zero harm.

Questions for Discussion

Q1: What is the main content of occupational hazards?

Q2: What problems and challenges have emerged in occupational prevention?

Text A

Occupational Health

Occupational Hazards

Occupational **hazard** factors, also known as occupational hazards, are factors or conditions that are generated and/or present in occupational activities that may adversely affect the health, safety, and work ability of workers. Occupational hazard factors can be divided by source into those related to the production process, those generated in the working process, and those which are **inherent** in the production environment. They can also be classified by nature into chemical, physical, biological, and human factors.

(1) Chemical occupational hazard factors: They include raw materials, intermediate products, and finished products, and waste gas, water, and residues generated in the production process, and other active factors to which workers are exposed in production and that can cause health hazards. Substances that are harmful to the human body when ingested even in small amounts are called **toxicants**. Toxicants often exist in the form of dust, smoke, mist, vapor, or gas. Once ingested, they can cause health effects, such as irritant contact dermatitis (ICD), neuropathy, liver damage, reproductive hazards, kidney damage, and respiratory, digestive, or cardiovascular abnormalities, etc. The main ways occupational chemical harmful factors invade the human body include: ① breathing (respiratory system), which is the most common way for harmful substances in the working environment to entering the body; air pollutants can be directly **absorbed** or **deposited** in the lungs, causing local irritation, or enter the blood to reach target organs, causing systemic diseases; ② skin contact; when the skin is injured, harmful substances can be quickly absorbed into the blood through the skin wound, whereas intact skin forms a barrier; however, some **fat-soluble** substances, such as **trinitrotoluene**, cyanide, **organophosphorus**, most **aromatic** amines, and **phenols**, are easily absorbed through intact skin, causing symptoms of systemic poisoning; and ③ ingestion (digestive system); in the workplace, workers may eat or drink harmful chemicals without knowing it; harmful substances are absorbed into the blood through the **gastrointestinal** tract, and then transported to other target organs, causing health hazards; for example, if workers eat, drink, or smoke in a workplace where lead is handled, they may accidentally ingest food contaminated with lead dust attached to their hands, thus causing serious health effects.

(2) Physical occupational hazard factors: Physical factors that cause health hazards in occupational activities often include **noise**, **vibration**, electromagnetic radiation, and adverse weather conditions, etc. Examples of such health hazards are hearing loss or physiological abnormalities caused by noise, vibration-induced white finger (VWF) caused by local vibration, caisson disease, high altitude disease, or altitude decompression sickness, etc., caused by abnormal air pressure, heat cramp, heat exhaustion, or heat stroke, etc., caused by high temperature **exposure**, **frostbite** caused by low temperature environment, skin lesions or eye damage caused by ultraviolet radiation, and skin burns and corneal inflammation caused by infrared radiation.

(3) Biological occupational hazard factors: Biological hazards in the workplace are caused by **pathogenic** bacteria, viruses, fungi, parasites, vector infections, animal and plant products, and their excreta, such as *Bacillus anthracis*, forest encephalitis virus, *Brucella*, *Borrelia burgdorferi* (causing Lyme disease), HIV, hepatitis virus.

(4) Ergonomic occupational hazards: Ergonomic occupational hazards include accidents or diseases in the workplace caused by poor design of plant layout, tools, and equipment, etc., or due to improper handling or lifting, poor visual conditions, uncomfortable postures, or repetitive actions, such as low back pain and **carpal** tunnel syndrome. Tools and workstations should be designed to be suitable for human use, taking into account human physiology, psychology, and biomechanics, so as to eliminate related health hazards.

(5) Occupational stress hazards: Occupational stress is a harmful physical and emotional reaction that occurs when work needs do not match personal abilities, resources, or needs. Occupational stress factors (social and psychological risk factors in the workplace) are work environment events or conditions that cause workers to produce such physical and emotional reactions. Studies have shown that occupational stress factors are related to cardiovascular disease, **musculoskeletal** system disorders, depression and other mental health problems, sleep disorders, job burnout, and suicide. Occupational stress factors are related to unhealthy lifestyles, such as excessive drinking, overweight, lack of exercise, and increased smoking, which increase health risks and affect the health of workers.

Occupational Health in China

The spectrum of occupational diseases in developed and developing countries is not the same, but occupational hazards are widespread. Inadequate occupational health services lead to a lack of necessary guarantees for sustainable development. It has become a common weak link in the development of economic globalization and a common obstacle in the development of occupational health globalization. Therefore, the WHO has clearly put forward the global strategy of "occupational health for all".

China is a country with the largest working population in the world. There are many kinds of occupational hazards, and occupational health has the characteristics of **hysteresis** and **potentiality**. Almost 200 million workers are exposed to various occupational hazards in China. Occupational disease is the result of the **interaction** between working conditions and the body. According to *the 2020 China Health Development Statistical Bulletin*, 14,408 new cases of occupational pneumoconiosis and other respiratory diseases were reported nationwide, and 6,668 deaths were reported due to pneumoconiosis. And there were also 488 cases of occupational infectious diseases, 486 cases of occupational poisoning, 217 cases of occupational diseases caused by physical factors, 63 cases of occupational skin diseases, 48 cases of occupational tumors were reported in 2020.

The occurrence of occupational diseases is closely related to the level of social productivity and the degree of economic development. While promoting global economic development, the integration process of the global economy will inevitably be accompanied by global health. Due to the increasing gap in the economic development level, there is a trend of occupational hazards transferring from abroad to home, from economically developed areas to economically backward areas, and from urban to rural areas. With the transformation and upgrading of China's economy, the emergence of various emerging industries such as the Internet, high-speed rail, aerospace and wind power has brought about the application of new processes, technologies, equipment and materials. For example, the rapid development of information technology, new renewable energy technology, biomedical technology, etc. The application of new materials includes the development and utilization of new chemicals, such as nanometer materials and the graphene industry. Workers are faced with new ways of operation and the subsequent surge of new occupational hazards. Such as occupational diseases caused to shift work assignments, mental health and occupational stress, improper posture load and ergonomics. All of these occupational hazards pose serious challenges to the health and safety of workers.

In addition to the traditional common occupational diseases such as pneumoconiosis, occupational poisoning and occupational noise-induced deafness, factors such as the aging labor population, mental illness, work-related musculoskeletal diseases and other factors lead to various chronic non-communicable diseases that have become the most urgent occupational health challenges. The damage of occupational psychology to health has been attracting much attention. Psychological load and mental fatigue is constantly aggravating among workers, producing occupational stress and other adverse psychological reactions. It may lead to sleep disorders and depression, thus increasing the risk of cardiovascular diseases and other diseases. Moreover, occupational hazards lead to a long incubation period of various chronic noncommunicable diseases, so the occurrence of many diseases is not at the career lifecycle. Exploring the long-term health effect of labor conditions is a very important research field and direction.

Future occupational health studies should value and establish **cohort** about occupational population. This is conducive to the etiology and prevention research, can find the law and evidence of occupational hazards. It can make a more complete explanation and clarification of the occurrence mechanism of occupational damage, to achieve early prevention. Secondly, pay attention to occupational health risk assessment. Through the multi-dimensional measurement of workers' psychological, behavioral, social and environmental factors, to identify the harmful factors and judge the possibility and severity of occupational hazards in work, so as to formulate corresponding measures. The assessment of external exposure can use automated environmental monitoring technology to automatically monitor the temperature, wind speed, and harmful gases of the individual surrounding environment, so as to realize real-time online monitoring and management of occupational hazards. Internal dose measurement methods such as the determination in blood and urine by inductively coupled plasma mass-spectrometry (ICP-MS), and the combination of liquid chromatography-mass spectrometry (LC-mass) and nuclear magnetic resonance technology to explore the value of diagnosis and prognosis of small molecule metabolites in occupational health damage. Fast-developing new molecular biology technologies and methods of high-resolution, large-throughput analysis of bioinformatics such as genomics, transcript-omics, proteomics, and metabolomics can all reflect the type and level of individual exposure from different perspectives. In addition, occupational health should effectively combine the advantages of evidence-based medicine, translational medicine and precision medicine. The study of occupational exposure and social sciences on the relationship between occupational exposure and health damage to protect and promote the health of occupational groups.

Words and Expressions

hazard 危险, 危害
*A new report suggests that chewing gum may be a health **hazard**.*

inherent 内在的,固有的

*When we use a substance, we must take into account the **inherent** properties of the substance.*

toxicant 毒药;有毒的

*There is no known antidote to the **toxicant**.*

absorb 吸收;使并入,纳入;同化,汲取;消减,缓冲;理解,掌握(信息);使全神贯注,使专心;承受(变革、影响等),承担(费用等)

*Plants **absorb** carbon dioxide from the air and moisture from the soil.*

deposit 沉积,沉淀;支付;放下,放置;储蓄;存放,寄存;沉积物,沉积层;订金;押金;存款

***Deposition** of respiratory dust in the lungs can cause pneumoconiosis.*

fat-soluble 脂溶性的,可溶于油脂的

*Vitamins can be classified into water-soluble vitamins and **fat-soluble** vitamins.*

trinitrotoluene (TNT) 三硝基甲苯;烈性炸药

*Exposure to **trinitrotoluene (TNT)** at work can cause lens damage in workers.*

Organophosphorus 有机磷

***Organophosphorus** poisoning is a common occupational poisoning in farmers.*

aromatic 芳香的,芬芳的;芳香族的;芳香植物;芳香剂

*Benzene is an **aromatic** compound.*

phenol 酚类,酚类化合物(phenol 的复数);[药]石炭酸

***Phenols** are the primary pollutant for human health.*

noise 噪声,嘈杂声

*There was too much **noise** in the room and he needed peace.*

vibration 震动,颤动,抖动

***Vibration** often springs many parts of the bike.*

exposure 暴露,接触;曝光,揭发;报道,宣传;朝向

*Their cancers are not so clearly tied to radiation **exposure**.*

frostbite 冻伤,冻;冻伤,遭受霜冻;冬季帆船比赛的

*Working in low temperatures for long periods of time can cause **frostbite**.*

pathogenic 致病的;病原的;发病的

***Pathogenic** agents such as fungi and bacteria can cause diseases in humans and animals.*

carpal 腕关节;腕关节的

*The main hand -related occupational hazard is **carpal** tunnel syndrome.*

musculoskeletal 肌(与)骨骼的

*Low back pain is one of the most common and costly **musculoskeletal** problems in modern society.*

hysteresis 迟滞现象;滞后作用

***Hysteresis** has historically been a bigger threat in the euro area than in America or Britain.*

potentiality 潜力,潜能;潜在性,可能性

*All of these are useful breeds whose **potentiality** has not been realized.*

interaction　互动, 交流; 相互影响, 相互作用

*One unpleasant **interaction** can have incidental effects on many other, unrelated judgments and decisions.*

cohort　一群; 队列

*During this prospective observational **cohort** study, about 2% of the men developed kidney stones.*

Language Points

occupational hazards　职业性有害因素

Factors or conditions produced and/or existing in occupational activities that may have adverse effects on the health and safety of occupational population, including chemical, physical and biological factors.

*At present, chemicals and dust are still the main **occupational hazards** in workplaces.*

occupational disease　职业病

Occupational practitioners of enterprises, institutions and individual economic organizations in occupational activities caused by exposure to dust, radioactive substances and other toxic and harmful factors.

There are ten categories of 132 kinds of legal occupational diseases in China.

irritant contact dermatitis (ICD)　刺激性接触性皮炎

Irritant contact dermatitis is an inflammation of the skin that does not produce specific antibodies.

*Occupational contact dermatitis can be divided into **irritant contact dermatitis (ICD)** and allergic contact dermatitis (ACD).*

electromagnetic radiation　电磁辐射

Electromagnetic radiation (EM radiation or EMR) is a form of radiant energy released by certain electromagnetic processes.

*What we are seeing from earth is actually **electromagnetic radiation** that comes from stars.*

vibration-induced white finger (VWF)　振动性白指

Vibration-induced white finger is a condition typically manifested by hand-arm vibration, also known as occupational Reynolds phenomenon.

VWF is easy to appear after a cold on the hands or whole body.

heat stroke　热射病

Heat stroke is a symptom mainly caused by central thermoregulation and sweat gland failure. The main features are headache, dizziness, thirst, hyperhidrosis and weakness of limbs.

*Working in high temperatures and low humidity for a long time is easy to suffer **heat stroke**.*

carpal tunnel syndrome　腕管综合征

Carpal tunnel syndrome is characterized by anterior wrist pain and hand numbness and weakness.

*The most famous injury caused by repetitive hand manipulation is **carpal tunnel syndrome**.*

nanometer materials　纳米材料

A new generation of materials made up of nanoparticles.

*The application prospect of **nanometer materials** was very wide.*

graphene　石墨烯

Electrons can flow through graphene with remarkable ease, making graphene an ideal material for transistors.

***Graphene** is pure carbon in the form of a very thin, nearly transparent sheet, one atom thick.*

shift work assignments　倒班作业

Shift work assignments is an organizational form of working time which needs workers to engage in work schedules on a rotational basis to maintain the uninterrupted operation of workplaces. *When introducing **shift work assignments,** the most important thing is to work out good work schedules.*

occupational stress　职业紧张

Occupational stress is stress involving work. According to the current World Health Organization's (WHO) definition, occupational or work-related stress "is the response people may have when presented with work demands and pressures that are not matched to their knowledge and abilities and which challenge their ability to cope".

*Working conflict was the main **occupational stress** factor.*

pneumoconiosis　尘肺

Pneumoconiosis is a group of occupational lung diseases caused by the long term inhalation of mineral, which leads to chronic pulmonary inflammation and fibrosis.

***Pneumoconiosis** is the most widespread and serious occupational disease, mainly characterized by pulmonary tissue fibrosis, and caused by long-term inhalation of productive dust in the production environment.*

occupational noise-induced deafness　职业性噪声聋

The first symptom of occupational noise deafness is hearing fatigue, which is a progressive sensorial hearing damage caused by long-term exposure to noise.

***Occupational noise-induced deafness** is one of the legal occupational diseases in China.*

work-related musculoskeletal diseases　工作相关肌肉骨骼疾患

It is commonly used to refer to a range of disorders, such as low back pain, arm vibration symptoms and carpal tunnel syndrome, that can be caused by a variety of occupational activities characterized by repetitive movements, long working hours, or forced positions.

***Work-related musculoskeletal disorders** can damage workers' health.*

incubation period　潜伏期

Incubation period is the time elapsed between exposure to a pathogenic organism, a chemical or radiation, and when symptoms and signs are first apparent.

*The **incubation period** is usually 3 to 14 days.*

career lifecycle　职业生命周期

The whole process from the beginning of a professional activity to complete withdrawal.

Career lifecycle is divided into four periods: exploration period, development period, stable period and decline period

occupational health risk assessment　职业健康风险评估

Occupational health risk assessment is a process in which occupational health risk level is evaluated qualitatively or quantitatively through comprehensive and systematic identification and analysis of workplace risk factors and protective measures, and corresponding control measures are taken.

Occupational health risk assessment is an important part of occupational health.

inductively coupled plasma mass spectrometry (ICP-MS)　电感耦合等离子体质谱法

Inductively coupled plasma mass spectrometry (ICP-MS) is a highly sensitive analytical technique which combines the high-temperature ionization characteristics of ICP with the advantages of sensitive and fast scanning of MASS spectrometer.

*The influence of different concentration of oxalic acid on elemental **inductively coupled plasma mass spectrometry** has been investigated.*

genomics　基因组学

Genomics is a discipline in genetics that applies recombinant DNA, DNA sequencing methods, and bioinformatics to sequence, assemble, and analyze the function and structure of genomes (the complete set of DNA within a single cell of an organism).

***Genomics** studies the function of genes, the DNA instructions by which the body makes proteins.*

transcriptomics　转录组学

The transcriptome is the set of all RNA molecules, including mRNA, rRNA, tRNA, and other non-coding RNA transcribed in one cell or a population of cells.

*It is thus widely used as an initial step for sequence characterization and annotation, phylogeny, genomics, **transcriptomics**, and proteomics studies.*

proteomics　蛋白质组学

Proteomics is the large-scale study of proteins, particularly their structures and functions.

*In the post-genomic era, **proteomics** has become the focus of research.*

metabonomics　代谢组学

Metabolomics is the scientific study of chemical processes involving metabolites. Specifically, metabolomics is the "systematic study of the unique chemical fingerprints that specific cellular processes leave behind", the study of their small-molecule metabolite profiles.

***Metabonomics** is a new branch of "-omics" science in post-gene time.*

precision medicine　精准医疗

Precision medicine (PM) is a medical model that proposes the customization of healthcare- with medical decisions, practices, and/or products being tailored to the individual patient. In this model, diagnostic testing is often employed for selecting appropriate and optimal therapies based on the context of a patient's genetic content or other molecular or cellular analysis.

***Precision medicine** will bring more new therapeutic strategies, drug discovery and development, and gene-oriented treatment.*

EXERCISES

Task 1: Vocabulary Application

Fill in the blanks with the words given below. Change the form where necessary.

liposoluble; occupational stress; density; noise; pneumoconiosis; vibration; gastrointestinal; hysteresis; pathogenic; organophosphorus

1. There was higher _____ in VDT work. It may have harmful effects on VDT operators' psychological health.

2. _____ and _____ are both of the important factors of physical occupational hazards.

3. Dose response relationship is an important method to evaluate toxicity and exposure _____ .

4. The rate of absorption through the skin is related to the _____ features of the substance itself.

5. _____ is one of the most common occupational diseases and there is no effective treatment.

6. Physical factors that cause health hazards in occupational activities often include noise, _____ , electromagnetic radiation, and adverse weather conditions, etc.

7. Workers may eat or drink harmful chemicals without knowing it; harmful substances are absorbed into the blood through the _____ tract, and then transported to other target organs, causing health hazards.

8. There are many kinds of occupational hazards, and occupational health has the characteristics of _____ and potentiality.

9. Biological hazards in the workplace are caused by _____ bacteria, viruses, fungi, parasites, vector infections, animal and plant products, and their excreta, such as *Bacillus anthracis*, forest encephalitis virus, *Brucella*, *Borrelia burgdorferi* (causing Lyme disease), HIV, hepatitis virus.

10. Some fat-soluble substances, such as trinitrotoluene, cyanide, _____ , most aromatic amines, and phenols, are easily absorbed through intact skin, causing symptoms of systemic poisoning.

Task 2: Writing

For this part, you are allowed 30 minutes to write a composition on the topic: occupational diseases. You should write at least 120 words, and base your composition on the outline below:

1) What harm will occupational diseases bring?

2) How to reduce the occurrence of occupational diseases?

Task 3: Oral Presentation

Occupational health work is an important part of health work. Under the background of the present era, occupational health work bears a new mission, and there should be new measures and new actions. Talk about your opinions on the main contents or measures of tertiary prevention in occupational health.

READING B

PREVIEW

Environmental hygiene focuses on exploring the relationship between the natural environment and the living environment and the health of the population. It is in order to reveal the occurrence and development of the influence of environmental factors on the health of the population, put forward health requirements and preventive countermeasures to make full use of the beneficial factors and control the harmful factors of the environment, and also improve human health and raise the health level of the whole population.

In current, environmental exposure is considered to be a main triggering factor of laryngitis, a common upper respiratory tract infection, especially in developing countries. However, unclear detrimental air pollutants and lack of understanding on the association between their early-life exposure and laryngitis warrant further investigation. Therefore, a retrospective cohort including 2328 preschool children was conducted during 2015–2016 in Shenzhen, China. Researchers measured ambient air quality of PM10, SO_2 and NO_2 at 12 monitoring stations, and obtained childhood laryngitis prevalence and confounding covariates by questionnaire. Multiple logistic regression analysis showed that the lifetime prevalence of childhood laryngitis (12.2%) was associated with an interquartile range increase in late preconception, prenatal and early-postnatal exposure to SO_2. Sensitivity analysis revealed that this relationship appeared more obvious among boys without parental atopy, mold/damp stains, or window condensate. Nevertheless, there was no relationship between early-life PM10 and NO_2 exposure and childhood laryngitis. These findings suggest that early-life exposure to SO_2 significantly increases the risk of childhood laryngitis. Preventive measures need to be implemented to mitigate industrial air pollution.

Questions for Discussion

Q1: Why did the author choose Shenzhen as the site to study the effects of air pollution on children?

Q2: What are the strengths and limitations of this study?

Text B

Effect of Preconception, Prenatal and Postnatal Exposure to Ambient Air Pollution on Laryngitis in Southern Chinese Children

Laryngitis is an acute upper respiratory tract infection (URTI) that can affect any part of the respiratory **mucosa**. The prevalence of childhood laryngitis in developing countries ($>$10%) is higher than that in developed countries ($<$10%). It is reported that Chinese children who have been diagnosed with URTI (i.e., laryngitis or **croup**) are commonly prescribed **antibiotics** during their early years. Hence, antibiotic use in early childhood is prevalent in China. Children diagnosed with URTI such as laryngitis and being treated with antibiotics for a long time are more likely to develop ear, nose and throat infections, **asthma** or other **allergic** diseases. Generally, URTI is related to both genetic and environmental factors. It is reported that laryngitis is mainly due to environmental exposure, as human genes do not change in a matter of decades. However, the main environmental factors contributing to laryngitis are still unclear, especially for children.

There is increasing evidence linking air pollution with URTI such as childhood laryngitis. Previous studies have found an obvious relation between traffic-related air pollution and childhood URTIs, including **bronchitis**, **otitis** media and upper airway **inflammatory** episodes. Typical air **pollutants** such as particulate matter$\leqslant$10 μm in diameter(PM10) and SO_2 are thought to be important factors contributing to the increased prevalence of sore throat, chronic **pharyngitis** and other acute respiratory infections. As the largest developing country in the world, China has undergone rapid urbanization and economic growth in recent decades. A huge amount of pollutants have been **discharged** from industrial **manufacturing** and vehicle exhaust, resulting in serious air pollution in China. In recent years, although some classical air pollutants such as PM10 and SO_2 have decreased in parts of cities due to the energy conservation and emissions reduction strategy conducted by the Chinese Government, the overall levels of air pollutants in many cities, especially in those with heavy industries, remain high.

URTI is a leading reason for hospital admission among preschool children. According to the Aguilera **hypothesis**, early-life exposure to certain environmental factors is likely to **exacerbate** URTI and the lower respiratory tract infections. However, most previous studies only focused on **postnatal** exposure to air pollutants. Studies concerning **prenatal** and **preconception** exposure to air pollutants are still limited. A recent study suggested that preconception, prenatal and postnatal exposure to air pollutants would lead to childhood allergic diseases and symptoms. However, whether these stages of early-life exposure to air pollutants may have adverse effects on URTI remains unclear, and **warrants** further investigation.

Shenzhen, located in the Pearl River Delta, is one of the most developed and urbanized regions in China. The rapid economic development in Shenzhen in recent decades has led to serious air pollution. According to the Seventh National Census of China, Shenzhen had a population of 17.53 million. It has a young population, with an average age of 33 years. Thus, it has a large number of children in kindergarten. However, data on children's early-life exposure to air pollutants and its relation to URTI is still limited.

Following up on the China, Children, Homes, Health Study conducted in 2010–2012 in several cities, a study in Shenzhen during 2015–2016 was conducted. Researchers proposed the hypothesis that early-life exposure to air pollutants may promote URTI development in children. The aim of this study was to investigate the impact of preconception, prenatal and postnatal exposure to air pollutants on childhood laryngitis.

A total of 4700 **questionnaires** were distributed to participating children from 30 kindergartens in Shenzhen, based on random selection and even distribution in the city. The questionnaire was designed in Chinese according to the International Study of Asthma and Allergies in Childhood with slight **modifications** considering the cultural and housing features of China for collecting information about personal health status, such as **preterm** birth and **gestational** age, possible chemical exposure at home, as well as family members' lifestyle. The questionnaire was completed by the parents, who were required to return the questionnaire to the kindergartens within one week.

Researchers observed a significant relationship between childhood laryngitis and exposure to SO_2 during late preconception and pregnancy. Childhood laryngitis exhibited a significant relationship with preconception SO_2 exposure during the month before conception. This relationship was not observed during the year before conception. In the multipollutant model, researchers observed significant *odds ratio (OR)* for exposure to SO_2 plus PM10, NO_2, and all three during the late preconception period. They found that childhood laryngitis was also significantly associated with prenatal exposure to the industrial air pollutant SO_2. This **correlation** was particularly strong during the first and third **trimesters**. They also found significant *OR*s for SO_2 during the first and third trimesters in the multipollutant model after adding other pollutants. Therefore, the *OR*s for before birth exposure to SO_2 were consistently significant.

Recent studies have revealed that prenatal exposure to SO_2 may cause URTIs such as otitis media, as observed in the study. Researchers also demonstrated that maternal exposure to ambient air pollution might make preschool children more **susceptible** to the common cold. Based on the Barker hypothesis, organs experience growth programming that is capable of disrupting development as well as changing gene **transcription** and expression on the premise of not changing the DNA **sequence**, thereby creating a phenotype that is more sensitive to air pollution, and leads to enduring susceptibility in later life. Although the preconception and prenatal periods are important, the effect of preconception exposure to the outdoor air pollution on childhood URTIs has never been investigated.

In the single-pollutant model, childhood laryngitis was significantly related to postnatal exposure to the industrial air pollutant SO_2 during the first year after adjusting for the **covariates**, but was not related to the past year. There was no relationship between laryngitis and exposure to PM10 or traffic-related air pollutant NO_2 during any window. Researchers also found significant *OR*s for SO_2 during the first year in the multipollutant model after adding other pollutants. Thus, the *OR*s for SO_2 exposure during the first year were consistently significant. This study further demonstrated that being exposed to SO_2 during the first year after birth could lead to childhood laryngitis. Children's exposure to environmental factors after the first year of birth can easily impair their respiratory and immune systems. Mounting evidence suggests the significance of postnatal exposure to ambient air pollution for the later development of childhood respiratory health.

Laryngitis risk due to SO_2 exposure during the late preconception period, first and last trimesters or throughout pregnancy, and first postnatal year were higher in boys, without parental

atopy, without **mold/damp** stains, and without window **condensation**.

SO$_2$ is a highly **water-soluble** and **irritating** gas that is mainly from industrial coal and fossil fuel emissions, and could be an important cause of human respiratory diseases and serious air pollution. SO$_2$ can be absorbed by wet mucous **membranes**, generating **sulfuric** acid and **sulfite** as it passes through the respiratory tract. Exposure to high concentrations of SO$_2$ can cause mucosal injury and a series of clinical symptoms. However, many studies have suggested that early-life exposure to SO$_2$, combined with other air pollutants like PM10 and NO$_2$, can make children susceptible to URTIs. Therefore, the problem of environmental quality urgently needs our attention. Developing new energy sources and improving coal-burning technology should be carried out as soon as possible.

This prospective cohort study is the first to investigate the effect of early-life exposure to air pollution on childhood laryngitis. This was a relatively large-sample study, and researchers specifically divided early-life exposure into three timing windows, which ensured the reliability and consistency of the results. The study also had some limitations. First, the answers to the questionnaire were based on the respondents' memories and indoor environmental factors were mainly from the questionnaire survey, which may have involved recall bias. Besides, families traveling and moving could result in exposure misclassification. Second, the study calculated children's exposure based on air pollutant concentrations in kindergartens but not at home or in the workplace. Third, an **inverse** distance weighted method was adopted for modeling the exposure to air pollution using the data obtained by the monitoring stations for ambient air quality, which might have resulted in exposure bias due to the small number of monitoring stations and the unclear air pollution source and condition for land use.

Words and Expressions

laryngitis 喉炎

*In others, excessive smoking, or occupational pollution, cause metaplastic changes which alter the lining of the larynx enough to be diagnosed as chronic **laryngitis**.*

mucosa 黏膜

*Infection is often located on oral mucosa and respiratory tract **mucosa**.*

croup 格鲁布性喉头炎，哮吼

***Croup** is usually caused by a viral infection, and can be the result of a number of different viruses.*

antibiotic 抗生素

***Antibiotics** should be used to clear up the infection.*

asthma 哮喘，气喘

*The drug is set to become the treatment of choice for **asthma** worldwide.*

allergic 对……过敏的，过敏引起的，过敏性的

*Many people are **allergic** to airborne pollutants such as pollen.*

bronchitis 支气管炎

*An increase in some cancers and **bronchitis** may reflect changing smoking habits and poorer air quality, say the researchers.*

otitis 耳炎

*Studies show treating **otitis** with antibiotics leads to more ear problems.*

inflammatory 炎症性的

*That is, the bodies of these happy people are preparing them for bacterial threats by activating the pro-**inflammatory** response.*

pollutant 污染物

*Sulphur dioxide is a **pollutant** and a major contributor to acid rain.*

pharyngitis 咽炎

*Hemophilus influenzae accounted for 65% of the pathogenic bacteria in acute **pharyngitis**.*

manufacture 批量生产, 制造业

*There are many procedures involved in the **manufacture** of food that result in greenhouse gases and other pollutants.*

hypothesis 假说

*The statistics to prove or disprove his **hypothesis** will take years to collect.*

exacerbate 使加剧, 使恶化

*He also warned that global warming could **exacerbate** the problem by causing drought.*

postnatal 产后的

*All women in the province can avail of pregnancy and **postnatal** services through the Regional Health Authorities.*

prenatal 产前的

*Gestational diabetes is most often diagnosed through **prenatal** screening, rather than reported symptoms.*

preconception 孕前

*Nutrition advice is considered an important component of the **preconception** care.*

warrant 使有必要, 值得

*The recommendations provided in the report **warrant** our careful study.*

questionnaire 问卷

*The **questionnaire** was administered by trained interviewers.*

modification 修改, 修饰

*These fears are mostly exaggerated: as with hysteria about genetic **modification**, we humans are generally wise enough to manage these problems with speed and care.*

preterm 早产地

***Preterm** birth is an important perinatal health problem across the globe.*

gestational 妊娠期的

*Maternal body mass index is a predictor of neonatal hypoglycemia in **gestational** diabetes mellitus.*

odds ratio (*OR*) 优势比, 比值比

*Ever-smokers had an **odds ratio** of Hodgkin lymphoma of 1.4 compared with nonsmokers,* *and for current smokers the OR was 1.7.*

correlation 相互关系，关联

*The **correlation** of carbon dioxide with temperature, of course, does not establish whether changes in atmospheric composition caused the warming and cooling trends or were caused by them.*

trimester 孕期

*At the end of the first **trimester**, the fetus is about three inches long.*

transcription 转录

*A second important **transcription** factor required for osteoblastic differentiation is osterix.*

sequence 序列

*At each location on the **sequence**, we can measure all these different attributes of chromatin.*

covariate 协变量

*The job may require an individual who understands the meaning of interim analyses, multiplicity, cross-over, non-inferiority, **covariate** and subpopulations.*

atopy 特异反应性

*This condition, known as **atopy**, is thought to occur anywhere from 30 to 50 percent of the general population.*

mold 霉菌

*A MERV rating tells you how well the filter can remove pollen and **mold** from the air as it passes through.*

damp 潮湿的

*The plants grow best in cool, **damp** conditions.*

condensation 凝结，凝聚反应

*One of the most powerful weather systems, hurricanes are powered by the heat energy released by the **condensation** of water vapor.*

water-soluble 能溶解于水的

*Nitrate and **water-soluble** organic nitrogen were migrated with deionised water migrating and increased subsoil fertility.*

irritate 刺激

*Some drugs can **irritate** the lining of the stomach.*

membrane 膜，细胞膜

*These are substances which specifically latch onto the protein on the cell **membrane**.*

sulfuric 硫黄的，含（六价）硫的

***Sulfuric** acid eats away at limestone very aggressively.*

sulfite 亚硫酸盐

*The inhibition of hydroquinone on **sulfite** oxidation was investigated by oxygen removal and air oxidation tests.*

inverse 相反的

*In 6% of the cases, an **inverse** distribution may occur, with rash mostly on the extremities.*

Language Point

upper respiratory tract infection (URTI)　上呼吸道感染

A respiratory tract infection affects the respiratory system, the part of your body responsible for breathing. These infections can affect your sinuses, throat, lungs or airways. There are two types of respiratory infections: upper respiratory infections, and lower respiratory infections. Upper respiratory tract infections can be defined as self-limited irritation and swelling of the upper airways with associated cough and no signs of pneumonia, in a patient with no other condition that would account for their symptoms, or with no history of chronic obstructive pulmonary disease, emphysema, or chronic bronchitis. Upper respiratory tract infections involve the nose, sinuses, pharynx, larynx, and large airways.

*The study found that modern medicine, dandelion treat **upper respiratory tract infection**, acute bronchitis, gastroenteritis and so on.*

particulate matter　颗粒物

Particulate matter is a generic term to classify air pollutants comprising suspended particles in air, varying in composition and size, resulting from various anthropogenic activities. Industrial facilities, power plants, vehicles, incinerators, dust and fires are the major sources of particulate matter. The particle size ranges between 2.5 mm (PM2.5) and 10 mm (PM10).

*The solid and liquid **particulate matter** emitted by man-made and natural sources could endanger health.*

prospective cohort study　前瞻性队列研究

An epidemiological study in which subjects are selected from a specific population and divided into groups based on current or past exposure to a factor to be studied. The subjects were followed up and observed for a period of time to check and grade the occurrence of expected outcomes in each group. Compare the incidence of each group to evaluate and validate the relationship between study factors and outcomes.

*We performed a multicenter, **prospective cohort study** of 102 patients co-infected with HIV and HBV who were treated with TDF.*

recall bias　回忆偏倚

Recall bias is a systematic error. Because participants interviewed in the study could not accurately recall previous events or experiences, or ignored some details in the events: the accuracy and capacity of memories may be affected by subsequent events and experiences. Recall bias is a problem in studies using self-reporting, such as case-control studies and retrospective cohort studies.

***Recall bias** happened because the study was retrospective rather than prospective.*

EXERCISES

Task 1: Vocabulary Application

Fill in the blanks with the words given below. Change the form where necessary.

antibiotic; allergy; preconception; cohort study; correlation; prenatal; transcription; otitis; covariance; modification; asthma

1. Until research provides better answers, though, the report advises taking effective measures now, such as screening women for known medical conditions that could put them at risk during pregnancy, assuring good nutrition before and during pregnancy, and making sure that all women have access to good _____ and _____ health care and receive the recommended number of visits during pregnancy.

2. The best option is usually no _____ at all, except in the case of acute _____ .

3. _____ illustrates the degree to which two variables vary with respect to each other, while _____ determines the strength and direction of this relationship.

4. During post- _____ _____ in eukaryotes, a 5 'cap and a 3' polytail are added and introns are spliced and this process does not exist in prokaryotes.

5. Frequently, sufferers of this kind of _____ are also sufferers of_____ .

Task 2: Writing

You have a social-media account with a lot of followers. In view of the serious air pollution, you hope everyone can make a contribution to protecting the environment. For this part, you are allowed to write a paragraph about the pollutants in the air and the harm they do and also call on people to care for the environment and reduce energy consumption. You should write at least 150 words but no more than 300 words.

Task 3: Oral Presentation

Have a debate under the title "Are human beings the destroyers or the protectors of the environment".

Learning Garden

Endocrine Disrupting Chemicals (EDCs)

Endocrine Disrupting Chemicals (EDCs), also known as environmental hormones, are exogenous chemicals that disrupt the endocrine system. They do not directly cause abnormal effects on organisms as other toxic environmental pollutants, but imitate the effects of biological hormones, thus destroying homeostasis and causing serious effects on the generation, release, transport and metabolism of natural hormones in the process of human development. Even if the human body is exposed to very small amounts, they can cause endocrine disorders and various abnormal symptoms. These substances can cause physical and human reproductive disorders, abnormal behavior, reduced reproductive capacity and infant death.

Most of the EDCs are organic pollutants and heavy metals, about 70%-80% of pesticides and most of the stabilizers and plasticizers in plastics are EDCs, such as alkyl phenol (AP), alkyl phenol polyoxyethylene ether (APE), bisphenol A, phthalate esters (PAE), polychlorinated biphenyls (PCB), organochlorine pesticides, etc.

（陈青松、陆少游）

Unit 5   Nutrition and Food Hygiene

READING A

PREVIEW

Noncommunicable diseases (NCDs), such as cardiovascular disease, cancer, chronic respiratory disease, and diabetes, are the leading causes of death worldwide and represent an emerging global health threat. Every year 15 million people die of NCDs before they're 70, with 86% of these premature deaths occurring in low-and middle-income countries. The Global Burden of Disease Study suggests that an unbalanced diet is a major risk factor in the prevalence of NCDs. An unbalanced diet is often characterized by a high consumption of carbohydrates, lipids or proteins, and a low intake of dietary fiber, as well as vitamins and minerals. Under the interconnected personal, community, sociocultural, national, and global determinants of food environments and choices, adherence to balanced diets is thus required to keep us away from NCDs.

Questions for Discussion

Q1: What is the significance of healthy dietary patterns for noncommunicable disease prevention?

Q2: What unhealthy dietary patterns are spreading among the Chinese population?

Text A

Let Food Be Your Noncommunicable Disease Medicine

The Global Burden of Disease Study (GBD) aims to measure disability and death from a multitude of causes worldwide. It has grown over the past three decades into an international consortium of nearly 5,500 researchers from 150 countries. The latest GBD report in 2019 has shown that noncommunicable diseases (NCDs), such as heart disease, **stroke**, cancer, and chronic respiratory disease, **continue** to be the leading cause of death worldwide. In China, home to a fifth of the global population, NCDs account for approximately 86.6% of total death. **Specifically**, the main causes of death-cardiovascular disease, cancer, and chronic respiratory disease-accounted for 79.4% of total deaths. The **mortality** rate was 271.8/10 million due to cardiovascular disease, 144.3/10 million due to cancer (the top five being **lung**, **liver**, **gastric**,

esophageal, and **colorectal** cancer), and 68/10 **million** due to chronic **respiratory** disease.

NCDs are of increasing concern to society and national government. Although the **pathogenesis** of NCDs remains largely unknown, it has been generally accepted that NCDs could be prevented by a reduction in these risk factors. The main risk factors for NCDs can be classified into the categories of genetic factors, environmental factors, factors of medical conditions, and socio-demographic factors. Among them, healthy diet is **essential** in managing the risk of NCDs at all stages of life. As they are of the utmost importance, we **highlight** some basic concepts and knowledge on the dietary role in NCDs.

Nutrition is the **biochemical** and **physiological** process through which an organism uses food to support its life. It encompasses **absorption**, **distribution**, **metabolism** and **excretion**. Proper **nutrition ensures** the development and maintenance of an organism's health at all stages of life, including **fetal** development in the mother's **womb**. The seven major classes of **relevant** nutrients for humans are carbohydrates, dietary fiber, lipids, proteins, minerals, vitamins, and water. Nutrients can be classified as either **macronutrients** (**carbohydrates**, dietary fiber, **lipids**, **proteins**, and water needed in gram quantities) or **micronutrients** (**vitamins** and **minerals** needed in milligram or microgram quantities).

Although diet and nutrition have been studied for centuries, modern nutritional science is surprisingly young. The first vitamin B_1 was isolated and chemically defined in 1926, less than 100 years ago, ushering in a half-century of discovery focused on single nutrient deficiency diseases. For example, deficiency of vitamin C, namely ascorbic acid, leads to **scurvy**. Early symptoms of scurvy typically include weakness, fatigue, and soreness in the arms and legs. Progressively, there may be a decrease in red blood cells, gum disease, changes to hair growth patterns, and bleeding from the skin. As scurvy worsens further, poor wound healing can occur along with personality changes and ultimately death due to infection or bleeding. Another example is iron deficiency **anemia**, a condition in which blood lacks adequate healthy red blood cells. Red blood cells are known to carry oxygen to the body's tissues. People with mild or moderate iron-deficiency anemia may not have any signs or symptoms. More severe iron-deficiency anemia may cause fatigue or tiredness, shortness of breath, or chest pain.

Apart from nutrient deficiency diseases, the role of malnutrition in NCDs, such as cardiovascular diseases, diabetes, obesity, and cancers, has received great attention since the 1950s. Excessive caloric intake, an imbalance among proteins, carbohydrates and lipids, lack of minerals, vitamins and dietary fiber, as well as excessive consumption of refined/processed foods have been associated with increased risks for NCDs worldwide. With the rapid development of the national economy in China, there have been profound changes in dietary patterns. These changes are characterized by a reduction in cereal and vegetable consumption and an increase in animal food and oil/fat consumption. Concomitantly, the major causes of disease and death in China have shifted from predominantly infectious diseases and nutrient-deficient diseases to overweight/obesity and other non-communicable diseases. Surprisingly, nutritional modulations targeting either single or complex nutrients often fail to affect the risks of NCDs, though they are successful in the prevention and/or treatment of nutrient-deficient diseases. Instead, a great number of studies have suggested that modifying dietary patterns rather than focusing on individual foods or nutrients is more effective at preventing NCDs. One central dietary pattern for preventing NCDs is the Mediterranean diet. The Mediterranean diet varies across countries and regions; therefore it does not have a standard definition. However, it typically includes high intakes of vegetables, fruits, legumes, nuts, beans, cereals, grains, fish, and olive oil while having low intakes of meat and dairy foods.

Like nutrition science, nutrition policy needs to move from simplistic, reductionist strategies to multifaceted approaches. Nutrition policy to control non-communicable diseases has so far generally relied on consumer knowledge-simply inform the public through education, dietary guidelines, product nutrition labels, etc., and people will make better choices. To be effective, future nutrition policy must unite modern scientific advances on evidenced-based dietary information with trusted communication to the public. This requires a shift from the global medicalization of health towards addressing the interconnected personal, community, sociocultural, national, and global determinants of food environments and choices. Fortunately, the Healthy China 2030 initiative has been conducted to spread healthy dietary patterns among the public for optimal health during all stages of life.

Words and Expressions

stroke　脑卒中

*A **stroke** is a medical condition in which poor blood flow to the brain causes brain cell death.*

continue　继续,连续,维持,持续

*The Mediterranean diet **continues** to be named the Best Overall Diet worldwide.*

cancer　癌症,恶性肿瘤

***Cancer** is a condition where cells in a specific part of the body grow and reproduce uncontrollably.*

specifically　特别地,明确地,具体地

*He is interested **specifically** in food science.*

lung　肺脏

*The **lungs** situated within the thoracic cavity of the chest are the primary organs of the respiratory system in humans. The major function of **lungs** is to help you breathe. In 2015, there were an estimated 733,000 new **lung** cancer cases (17% of total cancer incidence) and 610,000 deaths (21.7% of total cancer mortality) in China.*

liver　肝脏

*The **liver** that is the body's largest internal organ, has many functions in the body, including bio-synthesizing proteins and blood clotting factors, manufacturing triglycerides and cholesterol, glycogen synthesis, and bile production. In China, more than 78% of **liver** cancers are caused by chronic infection.*

gastric　胃的

*China is one of the countries with the highest incidence of **gastric** cancer, and accounts for* *over 40% of all new **gastric** cancer cases in the world.*

esophageal　食管的

*The esophagus is a muscular tube that connects the mouth and stomach. Smoking, heavy alcohol use, and high salt can increase the risk of esophageal cancer. Typical signs and symptoms of **esophageal** cancer are painful or difficult swallowing.*

colorectal　结直肠的

***Colorectal** cancer is the development of cancer from the colon or rectum (parts of the large intestine). Typical signs and symptoms may include blood in the stool, a change in bowel movements, weight loss, and fatigue. In China, **colorectal** cancer ranked fourth and fifth in the highest incidence and mortality rates of all malignancies in 2018.*

Million　百万

*In the world of wealth, nine **million** people die every year from hunger. Please do not waste your food.*

pathogenesis　致病原因

***Pathogenesis** is defined as the origination and development of a disease. For example, acquired immunodeficiency syndrome (AIDS) is caused by human immunodeficiency virus (HIV) infection.*

essential　本质的,关键的,重要的

*Being aware of what and how much we eat is **essential** to good health.*

highlight　强调,照亮,加亮,使突出

*Your article should **highlight** your original findings.*

biochemical　生物化学的

***Biochemical** science is the study of the chemical substances and vital processes occurring in live organisms.*

physiological　生理的

***Physiological** science is the study of how the human body works.*

absorption　吸收

*The small intestine is the main site of nutrient **absorption**.*

distribution　分布

*After absorption, nutrients and these metabolites undergo these **distribution** across tissues/organs.*

metabolism　代谢转化

*Nutrient **metabolism** defines the molecular fate of nutrients and other dietary compounds in an organism.*

nutrient　营养素

*The best way to get **nutrients** that our body needs is from natural foods but not nutrient supplements for a healthy population.*

ensure　担保;保证;使安全

*There are many different kinds of foods, which helps to **ensure** that people eating a well-balanced diet receive an adequate amount of essential nutrients.*

fetal　胎儿

*The nutritional status of women before and during pregnancy plays a key role in **fetal*** *growth and development.*

womb　子宫

*The **womb** (also namely uterus) is a pear-shaped organ where a baby is carried during pregnancy.*

relevant　相关的

*Curbing the global obesity epidemic requires a population-based, multisectoral, multidisciplinary, and culturally **relevant** approach.*

macronutrients　宏量营养素

*Carbohydrates, fat, and protein are called **macronutrients**, which are the nutritive components of food to provide energy to maintain the body's structure and systems.*

carbohydrate　碳水化合物

*A **carbohydrate** is a biomolecule consisting of carbon (C), hydrogen (H) and oxygen (O) atoms, usually with a hydrogen–oxygen atom ratio of 2:1 (as in water) and thus with the empirical formula $C_m(H_2O)_n$.*

lipids　脂质

***Lipids** are molecules that contain hydrocarbons and constitute the building blocks of the structure and function of living cells.*

protein　蛋白质

***Proteins** are made up of chemical 'building blocks' called amino acids.*

micronutrients.　微量营养素

*Vitamins and minerals are called **micronutrients**, which are nutritive components of food to regulate host metabolism to maintain the body's structure and systems.*

vitamin　维生素

*A **vitamin** is an organic molecule (or a set of molecules closely related chemically, i.e. vitamers) that is an essential micronutrient which an organism needs in small quantities for the proper functioning of its metabolism.*

mineral　矿物质

*In the context of nutrition, a **mineral** is a chemical element required as an essential nutrient by organisms to perform functions necessary for life, except for oxygen, hydrogen, carbon, and nitrogen.*

scurvy　坏血病

*James Lind is remembered as the man who helped to conquer a killer disease. His reported experiment on board a naval ship in 1747 showed that oranges and lemons were a cure for **scurvy**.*

anemia　贫血症

***Anemia** is a condition in which you lack enough healthy red blood cells to carry adequate oxygen to your body's tissues.*

Language Points

Global Burden of Disease Study　全球疾病负担研究

Global Burden of Disease Study (GBD) is a comprehensive regional and global research program of disease burden that assesses mortality and disability from major diseases, injuries, and risk factors.

*The **Global Burden of Disease Study (GBD)** is now produced by an active collaboration of over 8,000 scientists and analysts from more than 150 countries.*

noncommunicable diseases 慢性非传染性疾病

Noncommunicable diseases (NCDs), also known as chronic diseases, are not passed from person to person.

***Noncommunicable diseases (NCDs)** are a growing threat to children and adolescents. NCDs undermine children's and adolescents' right to health, nutrition, education and play. The risk factors for NCDs are behaviors established in childhood and adolescence.*

heart disease 心脏病

Heart disease refers to several types of conditions that affect the heart. Coronary artery disease, arrhythmia, heart valve disease, and heart failure are the four most common types of heart disease.

*Exercise tests help reveal how the heart responds to physical activity and whether **heart disease** symptoms occur during exercise. If you can't exercise, you might be given medications.*

dietary pattern 膳食模式

A dietary pattern is defined as the quantity, variety, or combination of different foods in a diet and the frequency with which they are habitually consumed.

*With rapid economic growth and urbanization, the Chinese **dietary pattern** has changed considerably in the past four decades, from a predominantly plant-based diet to one including large amounts of animal products, with less consumption of cereals and vegetables and more intake of red meat, processed meat, and sugar-sweetened beverages.*

EXERCISES

Task 1: Vocabulary Application

Fill in the blanks with the words given below. Change the form where necessary.

> anemia; ascorbic acid; communicable diseases; excess; macronutrients; Mediterranean diet; micronutrients; non-communicable diseases; nutrition; pathogenesis

1. Although several risk factors relevant to life styles for noncommunicable diseases have been uncovered, these _____ remains largely unknown.

2. The leading cause of death worldwide in the 21st century is _____ .

3. _____ is the biochemical and physiological process by which an organism uses food to support its life.

4. Carbohydrates, lipids and proteins are called _____ , which are the major nutrients in the common human diet.

5. Vitamins and minerals are _____ your body needs in small amounts to work properly and stay healthy.

6. Vitamin C is also called _____ .

7. For vegans, who give up all animal products including dairy, eggs, and even honey, _____ are prone to occur by heme iron deficiency.

8. _____ caloric intake is closely linked to the incidence of diabetes.

9. _____ has long been thought to be a heart-healthy eating pattern that includes the food staples of people who live in the countries around the Mediterranean Sea, such as Greece, Croatia, and Italy.

10. The major causes of disease and death in China have shifted from predominantly _____ and diet-related deficiency diseases to non-communicable diseases.

Task 2: Writing

For this part, you are allowed 30 minutes to write a composition on the topic: noncommunicable diseases. You should write at least 120 words, and base your composition on the outline below:

1) Noncommunicable diseases are the major cause of death worldwide.

2) What is the relationship between unhealthy diet and noncommunicable diseases?

3) What measures should we take to protect against noncommunicable diseases?

Task 3: Oral Presentation

China has the world's largest population, going under health transition due to industrialization, urbanization, and a sedentary lifestyle. Around 86.6% of China's disease burden is caused by noncommunicable diseases. Please provide some management and prevention strategies for noncommunicable diseases and their risk factors from the perspective of nutrition.

READING B

PREVIEW

Food safety and nutrition are inextricably linked to each other. Access to sufficient amounts of safe and nutritious foods is essential for life and health promotion. Many food safety problems, such as foodborne diseases, have been longstanding problems affecting human health throughout history. Foodborne diseases are mainly caused by contamination of food or water by harmful microorganisms or toxic chemicals and may occur at any point in the process from food production to consumption. Infants, young children, older adults, and sick individuals are more susceptible to foodborne diseases, leading to a vicious cycles of disease and malnutrition. Despite governments worldwide making efforts over the years to improve the safety of the food supply, the occurrence of foodborne diseases remains a significant public health challenge in both developed and developing countries, and they contribute significantly to global mortality. It has been estimated that nearly one in ten people worldwide fall ill after eating contaminated food each year, resulting in 420,000 deaths. Foodborne diseases also cause a considerable socioeconomic burden and harm tourism and trade. Most foodborne diseases are preventable with proper food preparation.

Task 1: Questions for Discussion

Q1: What are the relationships between nutrition and food safety?

Q2: Can you provide an example of food safety events that you have experienced or read from the news?

Text B

Foodborne Disease

According to the World Health Organization (WHO), foodborne diseases result from the **ingestion** of foods contaminated with harmful microorganisms or toxic chemicals. The contamination of food may occur at any stage of the food production, distribution and consumption chain, and can result from various forms of environmental contamination, including pollution in water, soil, or air, as well as unsafe food storage and processing. Foodborne diseases include not only **conventional** food poisoning, but also **enteric** infectious diseases, food-borne parasitic diseases, **zoonotic diseases**, **food allergies**, and chronic food poisoning caused by toxic and harmful pollutants in food.

Foodborne diseases are usually infectious or toxic in nature and caused by biological or chemical factors that enter the body via contaminated food or water. Biological factors include **bacteria** (such as *Salmonella*, *Campylobacter*, *Enterohaemorrhagic Escherichia coli* and *Listeria*), viruses (such as Norovirus), parasites (such as fish-borne trematodes), and prions. In addition to microorganisms, people also get sick from poisonous chemicals, including natural toxins (such as mycotoxins, marine biotoxins, cyanogenic glycosides, and toxins in poisonous mushrooms), heavy metals, environmental pollutants, residue of veterinary drugs, residue of **pesticides,** and improperly used food **additives**.

The most common symptoms of foodborne diseases are **gastrointestinal** symptoms, such as stomach pains, vomiting and diarrhea. Symptoms may occur very quickly after food consumption, or may take days or even weeks to appear. The duration and severity of symptoms depend on the cause of the disease. For most foodborne diseases, symptoms occur between 24-72 hours after eating contaminated food or drinking contaminated water. Foodborne diseases may also cause neurological, gynecological and immunological symptoms, systemic multiple organ failure and even cancer, resulting in long-lasting **disability** and even death. It is estimated that approximately 3% of foodborne disease cases may lead to long-term health problems. The consequences of foodborne diseases are usually more severe and more often **fatal** in susceptible populations, such as infants, pregnant women, older adults or sick individuals.

Foodborne disease is a growing public health problem all over the world. In 2015, WHO provided the first report on estimated burden of foodborne diseases caused by 31 pathogens, including bacteria, mycotoxins, viruses, parasites and chemicals at global and regional levels. It is estimated that 600 million people, or nearly one in ten people worldwide, suffer from foodborne diseases each year, resulting in 420,000 deaths. Children under the age of five account for almost 30% of deaths from foodborne diseases, with 125,000 deaths every year. Diarrheal diseases contribute to over half of all cases of foodborne illnesses affecting around 550 million individuals annually and causing approximately 230,000 deaths.

According to data collected from the National Foodborne Disease Outbreak Surveillance System in China, a total of 19,517 outbreaks of foodborne diseases were reported during 2003-2017, resulting in 235,754 illnesses, 107,470 **hospitalizations** and 1,457 deaths. The known **etiology** of 13,307 outbreaks was reported. Among these outbreaks, poisonous mushrooms accounted for 31.8% of outbreaks, followed by *Vibrio parahaemolyticus* (11.3%), saponin (8.0%), *Salmonella* (6.8%), **nitrite** (6.4%), pesticide (4.8%), *Staphylococcus aureus* (4.2%) and *Bacillus cereus* (3.0%). In terms of the locations where foodborne diseases occurred, 46.6% were associated with food prepared in households, followed by 22.5% with food prepared in restaurants and 18.4% with food prepared in canteens. Among the 13,305 outbreaks with known sources of contamination, **fungi** (mainly poisonous mushrooms) were the most common source, followed by meat, vegetables, aquatic animals, **condiments**, poisonous plants and grains.

Foodborne diseases not only have great impact on human health, but also cause a considerable burden on the economy, trade and even social stability. Countries all over the world have established foodborne disease **surveillance** systems to collect data on foodborne disease outbreaks and provide information on etiology, implicated food sources, settings, etc., in order to establish causal relationships between contaminated food and illnesses. International surveillance networks include WHO Global Salm-SUR, WHO GSS, FoodNet of the United States, EnterNet of the European Union. China has established a national foodborne pathogen surveillance network since 2000, which continuously and actively monitors *Salmonella*, *Enterohemorrhagic Escherichia coli* O_{157} : H_7, *Listeria monocytogenes* and *Campylobacter* in food. A foodborne disease surveillance network was established in 2002. In 2005, China established a surveillance program related to five enteric infectious diseases, including **dysentery**, **typhoid**/paratyphoid, **cholera**, *Yersinia enterocolitis* and *Escherichia coli* O_{157} : H_7 to monitor outbreaks, etiology, bacterial **resistance** and epidemic factors nationwide. In 2010, China began to establish a national reporting system for foodborne diseases (including food poisoning) and suspected foodborne abnormal cases or health events.

Food can become contaminated at any point in the process from production to consumption, and most foodborne diseases are preventable with proper food preparation. Since a large proportion of foodborne disease incidents occur in households, restaurants or canteens due to improper preparation or mishandling of foods, consumers and food handlers should be familiar with common food hazards and adopt basic hygienic practices to ensure food safety. WHO introduced Five Keys to Safer Food recommendations for safe food preparation, handling, and prevention of foodborne diseases. The core messages of the Five Keys to Safer Food recommendations are: keep clean, separate raw and cooked food, cook thoroughly, keep food at safe temperatures, and use safe water and raw materials.

Keeping clean is important because dangerous microorganisms are widely distributed in water, soil, animals and people and can easily be found on hands, wiping cloths, **utensils** and cutting boards. These microorganisms can be transferred to food or water through slight contact during food preparation and handling which may result in foodborne diseases. To maintain cleanliness, one should wash their hands before food handling, during food preparation and after going to the toilet. **Insects**, **pests** and other animals should be avoided to gain access to kitchen areas or food. All kitchen surfaces and equipment used for food preparation need to be washed and **sanitized** thoroughly following preparation.

Raw foods, especially meat, **poultry** and seafood, need to be separated from other foods because these raw foods and their juices may contain and transfer dangerous microorganisms onto other foods during food preparation and storage. People should use separate equipment and utensils such as knives and cutting boards for handling raw and cooked foods. Raw and cooked foods need to be stored in separate containers to avoid contact between each other.

Cooking food thoroughly, especially meat, poultry, eggs and seafood, to a temperature of at least 70℃ can kill almost all dangerous microorganisms and help ensure that the food is safe for consumption. To cook thoroughly, soups and stews should be heated until boiling point while meat and poultry should be cooked until their juices are clear rather than pink. It is ideal to use a thermometer when cooking, in order to monitor temperature change. Leftover food must always be reheated thoroughly before consumption.

Food should be stored at safe temperatures to slow down or prevent the growth of microorganisms. Cooked food should not be kept at room temperature for more than 2 hours. Instead, all cooked and **perishable** food needs to be promptly refrigerated (preferably below 5℃). However, it is important to note that several dangerous microorganisms can still grow below 5℃, so one should not store food in the refrigerator for too long. Refrigerated food should be cooked thoroughly and kept hot (more than 60℃) prior to serving.

Raw materials, such as water and ice, may be contaminated with dangerous microorganisms or poisonous chemicals. People should either use safe water or process the water to ensure its safety. Poisonous chemicals can form in damaged or **moldy** food, so it is necessary to carefully select fresh and wholesome foods that are within their expiration date or have been processed for safety, such as pasteurized milk. Fruits and vegetables should be washed thoroughly and peeled appropriately, especially if eaten raw.

Continued efforts are still required to reduce the incidence of foodborne diseases. Policy-makers can build and maintain strong systems and surveillance networks to manage food safety risks throughout the entire food chain from farm to processing plant, restaurants and households. Consumers and food handlers should be aware of common food hazards and can reduce foodborne disease risks by following recommendations to handle and prepare food safely.

Words and Expressions

inextricably　密不可分地；解不开地
*For these people, land is **inextricably** interwoven with life itself.*

contamination　污染

*It's not just dropping food on the floor that can lead to bacterial **contamination**.*

microorganism　微生物

*Animal faeces also contain **microorganisms** that can cause diarrhea.*

vicious　凶险的；严厉的；剧烈的

*The more pesticides are used, the more resistant the insects become, so the more pesticides have to be used. It's a **vicious** circle.*

ingestion　摄取；吸收；咽下

*Insufficient **ingestion** of staple food may thus impair memory.*

conventional　按照惯例的；习惯的

*Grass-fed milk can fetch up to 2.5 times the price of **conventional** milk.*

enteric　肠的，肠溶的

*These tablets are **enteric** coated and blister packed to prevent breakdown and inactivation of the ingredients.*

bacteria　细菌

*Warm milk is the ideal breeding ground for **bacteria**.*

pesticide　农药；杀虫剂

*Organic food is unadulterated food produced without artificial chemicals or **pesticides**.*

resistance　反对；阻力；抵抗力；免疫力

*AIDS lowers the body's **resistance** to infection.*

fatal　致命的；灾难性的

*This type of allergy can very occasionally be **fatal**.*

additive　添加剂，添加物

*Milk is sugar-free and **additive**-free with nutritionists recommending skimmed milk as the best choice before bed as it is the least fattening.*

poisoning　中毒

*In cases of food **poisoning**, young children are especially vulnerable.*

hospitalization　住院；住院治疗

*Infection was the most frequent cause of **hospitalization**.*

nitrite　亚硝酸盐

*Sodium **Nitrite** and Sodium Sulfite are additives used in food industry.*

fungi　真菌；菌类

*Ants can't digest the cellulose in leaves-but some **fungi** can.*

condiment　调味品，佐料

*Opt for grilled foods instead of fried, avoid or scrape away high-fat **condiments** like mayonnaise, and share those French fries to keep portion size down.*

dysentery　痢疾

*Some digging around in historical records revealed that there was a change in the incidence of water-borne disease at that time, especially **dysentery**.*

typhoid　伤寒

At an orientation meeting, the travelers were told that a visa, a landing card, and evidence *of inoculation against **typhoid** fever would be needed by each of them.*

cholera 霍乱

***Cholera** is a bacterial infection.*

utensil 餐具；炊具

*The doctor checks whether the **utensils** are clean enough for eating.*

insect 昆虫

*Honeybees use one of the most sophisticated communication systems of any **insect**.*

pest 害虫

*Each year, ten percent of the crop is lost to a **pest** called corn rootworm.*

sanitize 消毒

*Maintain clean and **sanitized** food preparation areas, to include all production equipment.*

poultry 家禽；家禽肉

*Contaminants found in **poultry** will also be found in their eggs.*

perishable 易腐烂的，易变质的

***Perishable** food should be stored in a refrigerator.*

moldy 发霉的；陈腐的，过时的

*Foods may become **moldy** easily on humid days.*

pasteurized 巴氏消毒的

*Using milk that has not been **pasteurized** can be dangerous.*

Language Point

food safety 食品安全

Food safety is a scientific discipline describing handling, preparation and storage of food in ways that prevent foodborne illness. This includes a number of routines that should be followed to avoid potentially severe health hazards.

*If people are suspicious of **food safety**, they will easily lose trust in the country.*

foodborne disease 食源性疾病

Poisoning or infectious diseases caused by the entry of pathogenic substances into the human body by means of food transmission

*The detection of foodborne bacterial pathogens is a key technological link for preventing and controlling **foodborne diseases**.*

food allergy 食物过敏

Allergic reaction to a substance ingested in food

*With the increase of age, **food allergy** reactions decreased, inhalation allergy reactions increased.*

*Markets crowded with domestic animals or wildlife are the perfect breeding ground for the spread of **zoonotic diseases**.*

EXERCISES

Task 1: Vocabulary Application

Fill in the blanks with the words given below. Change the form where necessary.

fatal; perishable; additives; ingestion; susceptible; bacterial; contamination; gastrointestinal; pasteurized; foodborne

1. The _____ of food may occur at any stage of the food production, distribution and consumption chain.

2. Salt intake may lead to raised blood pressure in _____ adults.

3. Insufficient _____ of staple food may impair memory.

4. The detections of _____ pathogens are the key technological link for the _____ disease prevention and control.

5. The most common symptoms of these diseases are _____ symptoms, such as stomach pains, vomiting and diarrhea.

6. This type of allergy can very occasionally be _____ .

7. Sodium nitrite and sodium sulfite are _____ used in food industry.

8. All cooked and _____ food need to be stored in a refrigerator promptly.

9. Using milk that has not been _____ can be dangerous.

Task 2: Writing

Unsafe food has been a human health problem since the beginning of recorded history, and many food safety problems encountered today are not new. For this part, you can write 2-3 tips that can help us prevent from foodborne diseases in daily life. You should write at least 150 words but no more than 300 words.

Task 3: Oral Presentation

For this part, you are allowed to talk about common foodborne disease contaminants in daily life, and please share one of your own experiences of infection with foodborne diseases. This oral presentation should be about 8 minutes long.

Learning Garden

Dietary Phytochemicals: Natural Swords Combating Noncommunicable Diseases

Phytonutrients handle important tasks in the secondary metabolism of plants as repellents to pests and sunlight as well as growth regulators. These compounds can be found in vegetables, fruits, beans, grains, nuts and seeds and are important components of the human diet. Phytonutrients aren't essential for keeping human beings alive, unlike the macronutrients and micronutrients that plant-derived foods contain. However, when consumed from plant-derived foods, phytonutrients help prevent and even treat diseases, especially noncommunicable diseases. Unexpectedly, most if not all human studies conducted so far have suggested that no individual or combination of purified phytonutrients can efficiently keep you away from noncommunicable diseases. Instead, we may obtain the most protection by eating a variety of plant foods rich in phytonutrients.

（孟荟萃、王冬亮）

Unit 6 Maternal, Child and Adolescent Health

READING A

PREVIEW

Maternal and child health (MCH) programs focus on health issues concerning women, children and families, such as access to recommended prenatal and well-child care, prevention of infant and maternal mortality, promotion of maternal and child mental health, newborn screening, child immunizations, child nutrition, and services for children with special healthcare needs. States invest in healthy children and families to strengthen communities and avoid unnecessary healthcare costs. Childhood and adolescence are critical periods for growth and development. Since the reform and opening up in China, the health conditions of children and adolescents have greatly improved. Meantime, data from the National Student Physical Health Survey have shown some problems for children and adolescents, such as high prevalence of myopia, overweight and obesity, as well as suboptimal physical fitness. The causes are believed to be mainly related to an unhealthy living environment, dietary styles, insufficient physical activities (especially outdoor activities), and excessive screen time. Therefore, society, schools, and families should create an excellent early family education environment, establish a social atmosphere of comprehensive education, healthy growth, and individualized development to ensure the health conditions of children and adolescents.

Questions for Discussion

Q1: What is the significance of public health for disease prevention in children and adolescents?

Q2: If you want to investigate the growth and development of local children and adolescents, what should be included in the survey plan?

Text A

Access to fruit and vegetable markets and childhood obesity

Obesity is a leading cause of **morbidity** and premature mortality, and the **prevalence** of overweight and obesity is increasing worldwide. From 1980 to 2013, the combined prevalence of overweight and obesity has risen by 27.5% for adults and 47.1% for children. The number of overweight and obese individuals has increased from 921 million in 1980 to 2.1 billion in 2013.

In particular, from 1975 to 2016, the global age-standardized mean **body mass index (BMI)** increased by an average of 0.32 kg/m^2 per decade for girls and by an average of 0.40 kg/m^2 per decade for boys. **Childhood obesity** is widely recognized as promoting the initiation and development of many **chronic** disorders such as **metabolic syndrome**, cardiovascular disease, and **diabetes mellitus**; it also increases the risk for adverse **psychosocial** consequences while lowering **educational attainment**. Since it is much more difficult to treat adulthood obesity, creating initiatives to prevent and **mitigate** childhood obesity is considered as one of the major **public health** challenges of the 21st century.

The **interaction** between the neighborhood environment and personal characteristics affects an individual's weight status. Some studies have examined how the **availability**, **accessibility**, **affordability**, **acceptability**, and **accommodation** of food in the neighborhood food environment influence **health-related behaviors** and weight gain. Fruit and vegetable markets (FVMs) are are crucial venues for providing healthy foods, as they often contain low energy and high **dietary** fibre content. Increased consumption of fruits and vegetables has been associated with the increasing satiety effect, which may play a critical role in preventing overweight and obesity. Children and adolescents are vulnerable to being influenced by their food environment as well as food marketing. Additionally, the lack of access to FVMs is thought to be a risk factor for childhood obesity because it discourages healthy dietary habits while promoting access to venues that offer more unhealthy food (and thus the compensatory intake of those options). Therefore, it is necessary to improve children's exposure to healthy food environments in order to protect them from the risk of developing obesity. The World Health Organization (WHO) has also emphasized the need for initiatives aimed at making fruits and vegetables more accessible in **residential neighborhoods**.

Access to certain types of food stores has been widely considered to contribute to childhood obesity, as children have limited control over their food choices during the **transition** to adolescence. However, here is no consensus on how much buffer zone distance between food stores and home or school could affect childhood obesity. Children and adolescents do not have unfettered access to private motorized travel, so a network buffer with a 0.8-km radius may better reflect a walkable distance for children, and they are more likely to be exposed to or become aware of available FVMs on their way home or to school. Long-lasting exposure to healthy foods increases the visibility of those foods, and as a result, children living in such environments may be more likely to accept and prefer healthy foods. However, results on the association between access to FVMs and childhood obesity are generally **inconsistent**. For example, six studies included in the systematic review reported no association between FVMs access and risk for overweight or obesity, five reported a negative association, and only one reported a positive association. The possible explanations include: ① access to fruit and vegetables is **ubiquitous**, and food shoppers are mobile, so measuring the density of FVMs and/or the distance to the nearest FVMs in the neighborhood may not reflect the actual accessibility of such healthy foods; ② other factors related to obesity and food purchase choices by children may be not be considered in the analyses, such as cultural factors, mobility, and access to public transportation.

Although some studies have reported associations between food environments, dietary behaviors and obesity, a critical approach is purchasing behaviors. Children may eat meals at home and/or school, and they may not make the food purchase choices as often by themselves as adults do. Thus, the availability of fresh fruits and vegetables around children's homes/schools may not affect their dietary behaviors and weight status. Instead, adolescents may be more likely to make food purchase choices.

Currently, studies have revealed no associations between the availability and accessibility of FVMs and weight-related behaviors and outcomes among children and adolescents. Nonetheless, it has important implications for future research and practice. Firstly, given that included studies used different terms to refer to FVMs and independently estimated FVM variables, further studies should provide clearer and more standardized definitions of FVMs to evaluate the effect of FVMs on child obesity more effectively. Second, the food environment is one of the most important **social determinants** of child obesity and influences health and obesity **disparities**. Therefore, further research should be carried out to understand the impact of the accessibility and availability of FVMs on childhood obesity.

Words and Expressions

obesity　肥胖；肥胖症

Obesity is a major risk factor of cardiovascular disease.

mitigate　减轻；缓和

Exercise could mitigate the psychological stress.

prevalence　流行

*Despite its **prevalence**, schizophrenia has existed behind a wall of secrecy for years.*

adolescent　青少年；青春期的；不成熟的

Most biologists, nonetheless, are doubtful that this is a humanlike **adolescent** growth spurt.

psychosocial　社会心理的

*The lack of **psychosocial** care reduces the effectiveness of the treatment.*

availability　可用性，可得性

*The nature and **availability** of material evidence was not to be discussed.*

accessibility　（地方）易于进入性，（物品）易于接近性

*In other words, Voltaire's amateurism in science "was a source of his contemporary appeal, demonstrating for the first time the **accessibility** of Newton's ideas to nonspecialists".*

affordability　可购性，负担能力

*Indeed, the emphasis on **affordability** might be slightly misplaced.*

acceptability　可接受性

*This assumption played a considerable part in increasing the social **acceptability** of divorce.*

accommodation　住宿

*The **accommodation** is simple but spacious.*

dietary　饮食的；有关饮食的；食谱；规定的食物

*After weighing the evidence, we can now confidently state that consuming pasta as part of a healthy **dietary** pattern does not have an adverse effect on body weight outcomes.*

transition　过渡，转变；

*The **transition** from school to work can be difficult.*

inconsistent　不一致的，不协调的，前后矛盾的

*The evidence given in court was **inconsistent** with what he had previously told them.*

ubiquitous　普遍存在的，无所不在的

*"I can envision a future in which robotic devices will become a nearly **ubiquitous** part of our day-to-day lives," says Gates.*

determinant　决定因素；决定条件；决定性的

*Even if precisely measured, income data exclude important **determinants** of economic well-being, such as the hours of work needed to earn that income.*

disparity　差距；（尤指因不公正对待引起的）不同，不等，差异，悬殊

*Research on the Economic **Disparity** and Impact Factor in Western China.*

Language Points

health-related behavior　健康相关行为

Health-related behavior is any overt behavior or personal attribute that either enhances or damages physical, psychological and social wellbeing now and in the future, even when heredity or environment is a negative factor and vice-versa.

*This survey collected information on **health-related behaviors.***

social determinants of health　健康社会决定因素

Social determinants of health (SDOH) are the conditions in the environments where people are born, live, learn, work, play, worship, and age that affect a wide range of health, functioning, and quality-of-life outcomes and risks.

***Social determinants of health** should be considered when assessing factors associated with health.*

BMI, body mass index　身体质量指数

Body mass index is a simple calculation using a person's height and weight. The formula is $BMI = weight (kg)/height (m)^2$ where kg is a person's weight in kilograms and m^2 is their height in metres squared. A BMI of 24.0 or more is considered overweight, while the healthy range is 18.5 to 23.9 (Chinese standard for obesity BMI).

*It is unhealthy to have either a very low or very high **body mass index.***

metabolic syndrome　代谢综合征

Metabolic syndrome is a disorder of energy utilization and storage, diagnosed by a co-occurrence of three out of five of the following medical conditions: abdominal (central) obesity, elevated blood pressure, elevated fasting plasma glucose, high serum triglycerides, and low high-density cholesterol (HDL) levels. Metabolic syndrome increases the risk of developing cardiovascular disease, particularly heart failure, and diabetes.

*People with **metabolic syndrome** need to go through a series of treatment.*

cardiovascular disease　心血管疾病

Cardiovascular disease is a class of diseases that involve the heart, the blood vessels (arteries, capillaries, and veins) or both. Cardiovascular disease refers to any disease that affects the cardiovascular system, principally cardiac disease, vascular diseases of the brain and kidney, and peripheral arterial disease. The causes of cardiovascular disease are diverse but atherosclerosis and hypertension are the most common.

*The prevalence of **cardiovascular diseases** are on the rise in many countries.*

diabetes mellitus　糖尿病

Diabetes mellitus (DM), commonly referred to as diabetes, is a group of metabolic diseases in which there are high blood sugar levels over a prolonged period. Symptoms of high blood sugar include frequent urination, increased thirst, and increased hunger.

*Many randomized controlled trials have tested new drugs that treat **diabetes mellitus.***

residential neighborhoods　住宅小区

Residential neighborhood means an area zoned residential, or a platted subdivision having two or more residences used for residential purposes.

*There are quite a few convenient stores around the **residential neighborhoods**.*

childhood obesity　儿童肥胖症

Childhood obesity is a serious medical condition that affects children and adolescents. It's particularly troubling because the extra pounds often start children on the path to health problems that were once considered adult problems-diabetes, high blood pressure and high cholesterol. Childhood obesity can also lead to poor self-esteem and depression.

Childhood obesity is more common than that in last century.

public health　公共卫生

Public health is the science of protecting and improving the health of people and their communities. This work is achieved by promoting healthy lifestyles, researching disease and injury prevention, and detecting, preventing and responding to infectious diseases. Overall, public health is concerned with protecting the health of entire populations. These populations can be as small as a local neighborhood, or as big as an entire country or region of the world.

*Most students majoring in preventive medicine eventually work in **public health** institutions after graduation.*

educational attainment　教育程度

Educational attainment refers to the highest level of education that an individual has completed. It is an important factor in determining whether people perceive a need for and seek urgent care.

*The average **educational attainment** of people living in country A is much higher than that in country B.*

EXERCISES

Task 1: Vocabulary Application

Fill in the blanks with the words given below. Change the form where necessary.

obesity; chronic; dietary; determinant; psychosocial; disparity; prevalence; accommodation; inconsistent; interaction; availability; accessibility; cardiovascular; morbidity; mortality; acceptability; transition; adolescents; affordability; ubiquitous

1. The study also demonstrated a direct link between _____ and mortality.

2. The illness frequently coexists with other _____ diseases.

3. Many mental disorders can be treated using _____ methods.

4. The increasing _____ of free access at hotels seems to be at a tipping point.

5. Consider the _____ in the relative chunks of income that go towards food and drink.

6. Fats and sugar are very rich in energy but poor in vitamins, minerals and _____ fibre, and they are associated with _____ .

7. Preterm birth and low birth weight (lbw) are major _____ of infant morbidity and mortality.

8. In the industrialized world, _____ diseases are the major cause of death.

9. This disorder is characterized by interlinking problems with social imagination, social communication and social _____ .

10. One study investigated how drug sample _____ affected what physicians prescribe.

Task 2: Writing

For this part, you are allowed 30 minutes to write a composition on the topic: Child and Adolescent Health. You should write at least 150 words and base your composition on the outline below:

1) Based on the health dimension, the index system and the life course view of health.

2) Discuss the main health problems and prevention of Chinese children and adolescents in recent years.

3) Explain the significance of health promotion in children and adolescents.

Task 3: Oral Presentation

In recent years, China has paid more and more attention to the problem of obesity in children and adolescents. Review the literature, analyze the reasons for the increase of obesity rate among children and adolescents in China, and select one of the three factors of "diet, exercise or sleep" to discuss its role and possible mechanism in the occurrence of obesity in children and adolescents.

READING B

PREVIEW

*Life history theory argues that unpredictable and harsh conditions such as early life adversity tend to produce a fast life history strategy, characterized by early sexual **maturation** and less parenting of offspring. It remains unclear whether all forms of early life adversity are* *associated with an accelerated reproductive strategy. Life history theory posits that individuals will select different allocation strategies according to the environment and life events experienced when resources are limited, trade-off physical growth and reproduction, so that resources and energy may be optimally allocated. Unpredictable and harsh conditions such as early life adversity (ELA) tend to produce fast life history strategy among women, characterized by earlier age at sexual maturation, earlier age at first birth, earlier age at **menopause**, and increased number of offspring. It remains unclear whether all forms of early life adversity are associated with accelerated reproductive strategy, and most previous studies predominantly focused on single form of reproductive strategy indicators.*

Questions for Discussion

Q1: What is life history theory?

Q2: What is the significance of accelerated reproductive strategy for middle-age women in China?

Text B

Associations between distinct dimensions of early life adversity and accelerated reproductive strategy among middle-aged women

Sexual maturity indicates the transition of energy expenditure from somatic growth to reproductive effort. Previous studies have reported the relationships among various types of early life adversity (ELA) and earlier age at **menarche** and menopause, including sexual abuse, **maternal** and **paternal** overprotection, family **dynamics** (e.g., parental divorce), and parental mental illness. However, little evidence is available on the associations of ELA with indicators of reproductive success (fitness), for example, the number of offspring and abortions. Research indicates that ELA is associated with an earlier age at first birth, and childhood experiences of physical and sexual abuse are individually associated with an increased risk of **miscarriage**. In general, most research to date has focused on single forms of reproduction strategy indicators; therefore, they were limited in their ability to capture the overall picture of reproductive timing and success.

It is important to acknowledge that these trends of ELA and faster life history are not universal. Life history-related traits seem to covary along a dimension of slow vs fast life history, reflecting the different trade-offs that individuals face in different environmental contexts. The **evolutionary** framework of life history theory predicts that the **diversity** of reproductive strategies in nature is shaped by environmental cues such as the resource scarcity (i.e., deprivation) and extrinsic **morbidity** and **mortality** (i.e., threat). In addition, recent conceptual models have emphasized the importance of distinguishing between threat-related ELA experiences characterized by environmental harshness (i.e., abuse and violent exposure) and deprivation-related ELA experiences characterized by the lack of expected environmental inputs (i.e., physical neglect, emotional neglect, and food insecurity). Findings from our studies and others have suggested that threat-related ELA was related to advanced age at **pubertal** onset, whereas no similar results were observed for deprivation-related ELA. Thus, the present study aims to identify and distinguish specific associations between ELA dimensions with indicators of reproductive timing, for example, age at menarche, menopause, and first birth, in addition to reproductive success, for example, number of offspring and **abortions**, in middle-aged women from the China Health and Retirement **Longitudinal** Study (CHARLS), which is a high quality nationally representative longitudinal survey of middle-aged residents in China, including assessments of social, economic and health status. The baseline national wave of CHARLS was conducted in 2011, and 3 follow-up surveys were carried out in 2013 (wave 2), 2015 (wave 3) and 2018 (wave 4), respectively. Further details about the CHARLS have been previously documented. Some researchers used data from the baseline (2011), 3 follow-up surveys (2013, 2015 and 2018) of CHARLS. The analytical sample was restricted to those women aged 40 and older at baseline and had information about ELA (n=9,674; mean [standard deviation] age at baseline, 55.89 [10.23] years).

Early Life Adversity Exposure

Multiple ELA experiences characterized by threat and **deprivation** were assessed using the Life History Survey Questionnaire in 2014. Participants were asked whether they experienced the specified adversities before the age of 17. Threat-related ELA included unsafe community dwelling, peer bullying, physical abuse from female or male **guardian**, being beaten by a **sibling,** and parental conflict; deprivation included absence of biological mother or father, food scarcity, poor family economic conditions, and loneliness.

Reproductive Strategy

Reproductive strategy outcomes were assessed from the follow-up of 2013, 2015 and 2018 via participant's recall and mainly included age at menarche (AAM), age at natural menopause (AANM), age at first birth, total number of children, and number of abortions (including spontaneous abortions, still birth, and induced abortions). The AAM, AANM, and age at first birth were collected at whole-year increments.

Principal Findings

In this national representative sample of middle-aged women in China, we found that a specific dimension of ELA (i.e., threat but not deprivation) was associated with aspects of a faster reproductive strategy. Greater exposure to ELA characterized by threat was associated with earlier AAM, natural menopause, and first birth along with an increased total number of children. In contrast, experiences of deprivation were associated with slower reproductive strategy indicated by a delayed age at menopause and increased number of abortions. This study is an extension of previous work, which demonstrates the specificity of ELA types and its associations with reproductive strategies.

Strengths

Evidence on the association between ELA and women's reproductive strategy from large well-characterized studies is scarce, compared with the data for this study, which comes from a large nationally representative longitudinal cohort study. In addition, researchers divided the ELA into two dimensions, threat and deprivation, and explored its association with overall reproductive strategy, which expands previous research.

Research Implications

A faster reproductive strategy includes less **prenatal** investment in individual offspring, which has been represented by lower birthweight and shorter **gestation** periods. Previous studies examining the associations between ELA and reproductive strategies rarely focused on **pregnancy** outcomes. Only one recent study suggested that ELA can result in reducing prenatal investment in individual offspring, characterized by shorter gestation period and higher offspring **cephalization** index. Future research should **incorporate** these indicators to provide evidence of a faster reproductive strategy extending to pregnancy outcomes. Although the specific dimension of ELA can accelerate reproductive strategy, it is not clear whether the acceleration is **pathologic** or adaptive. Researchers from Kenya used 48 years of longitudinal data from wild female baboons in the Amboseli ecosystem, and found that, although ELA led to shorter **lifespans** than those who did not experience ELA, individuals who experienced ELA did not accelerate their reproduction, and only long-lived baboons benefited from accelerated reproduction. In the future, it will be necessary to explore whether or not accelerated reproduction is an adaptive response to a specific early environment in humans.

Conclusion

A specific dimension of ELA (i.e., threat but not deprivation) was associated with accelerated reproductive strategy in the representative sample of middle-aged women in China and provides **preliminary** evidence of the effects of the different dimensions of ELA on reproduction. Future research should clarify the biological pathways between different dimensions of ELA and reproductive strategy and further determine whether accelerated reproduction is an adaptive response to early life adversity in humans.

Words and Expressions

maturation 成熟

*Finally, the enlightenment of relation between brain **maturation** and child behavioral development is discussed.*

menopause 绝经期;(妇女的)围绝经期

*Analysis on health care intervention of well-educated women in **menopause**.*

reproductive 生殖的;再生的;复制的

*Survey on **reproductive** health education and service demands of college students*

somatic 身体感觉;体细胞;躯体的;躯体

***Somatic** cells are produced from preexisting cells.*

menarche 初潮

*Young girls are very concerned about the time **menarche** and hope **menarche** time is normal.*

maternal　母亲的；母亲般慈爱的；母系的

Maternal age affects the baby's survival rate.

paternal　父系的；父亲的；慈父般的

*People have always focused on maternal age, but now we know that **paternal** age is also very important.*

dynamics　动力学；力学；动力；动态；演变；变革动力；力度变化；

*The interchange of ideas aids an understanding of family **dynamics**.*

abortions　堕胎；流产

*The World Health Organization estimates that 100, 000 women die each year from illegal back-street **abortions**.*

miscarriage　流产；小产；自然流产；流产；流产胎儿

*The 31-year-old, who was 17 weeks pregnant, died at University Hospital Galway following a **miscarriage**.*

evolutionary　进化的；进化论的；演化的；逐步发展的

*In **evolutionary** terms, this correlation may make sense.*

diversity　差异(性)；不同(点)；多样性；多样化

*Cultural **diversity** is a distinct characteristic of the world today.*

pubertal　青春期的

***Pubertal** period is a critical period for cognitive and behavioral development.*

longitudinal　纵向的，横断面的

*The Baltimore **Longitudinal** Study on Ageing followed the health of 1, 686 elderly people between 1980 and 1995.*

deprivation　缺乏；丧失；剥夺

*Sleep **deprivation** is an uncomfortable experience.*

guardian　保护者；保卫者；监护人

*A **guardian** of the person is entitled to regulate his education.*

sibling　兄弟姐妹

*Some studies have found that first-born children are more intelligent than their **siblings** born later.*

gestation　孕育期；怀孕期；妊娠期

*Clinical analysis of 20 cases of anomalous glucose metabolism during **gestation** period.*

pregnancy　怀孕；妊娠；孕期

*Drugs taken during **pregnancy** may cause physical deformity in babies.*

cephalization　头向集中，集头现象

*Recent study suggested that ELA can result in reducing prenatal investment in individual offspring, characterized by shorter gestation period and higher offspring **cephalization** index.*

incorporate　合并；包含；吸收

*We have **incorporated** all the latest safety features into the design.*

pathologic　病理的

*Critical evaluation of the effects of these changes on clinical and **pathologic** outcomes* *continues.*

lifespans　　寿命；使用期；有效期

*Different people may have different **lifespans**.*

preliminary　　预备性的；初步的；开始的

***Preliminary** studies showed that the instrument works well.*

Language Point

reproductive strategies　　繁殖策略

More recently, population genetics studies done by Blasco-Costa I have shown that host traits such as mobility can impact the spatial genetic structure of parasite populations, highlighting the potential evolutionary restrictions that hosts impose on parasite evolution in general and **reproductive strategy** in particular.

*The subject of demography has merged with that of the **reproductive strategies** of organisms.*

physical abuse　　身体虐待

The data from Colombian sample collected by Gavin Nobes indicates that the high rates of **physical abuse** by stepfathers resulted from numerous factors, perhaps beginning with parents' experience of abuse when they were children, and its subsequent intergenerational transmission via stressors such as interpersonal conflict and unstable relationships.

*Additionally, in the case of **physical abuse**, the only solution is to seek immediate help and shelter.*

sexual abuse　　性虐待

Sexual abuse is physical abuse that is physically or menacingly committed in order to satisfy sexual desire. Sexual abuse also includes sexual relations between the perpetrator and the child (under 18 years of age) in all circumstances.

*Childhood **sexual abuse** worldwide is a disturbing insidious offense with psychosocial impacts persisting into adulthood.*

spontaneous abortions　　自然流产

Spontaneous abortion refers to spontaneous termination of pregnancy before 28 weeks, with a fetal weight of less than 1000g. This definition is based on the World Health Organization's 1966 criteria for abortion.

*An increased risk of fetal death or **spontaneous abortions** in infected women has also been reported.*

still birth　　死胎

Fetal death in utero is the death of the fetus before the products of pregnancy are completely removed from the mother. Early fetal death is defined as occurring before 20 weeks of gestation, while middle and late fetal deaths are defined as occurring between 20-27 weeks and after 28 weeks of gestation, respectively. According to WHO, fetal death is defined as the absence of breathing or any other signs of life, such as heartbeat, umbilical cord pulsation, or definite voluntary muscle movement.

*A simple message that mothers could follow to reduce the risk of **still birth**, would be greatly appreciated.*

induced abortions　人工流产

Termination of pregnancy through artificial or medical means within the first three months of gestation is referred to as early termination of pregnancy, also known as induced abortion. It is used as a remedial measure for contraceptive failure and unintended pregnancies. It is also employed in cases when pregnancy would be detrimental due to disease or when termination is necessary to prevent congenital malformation or genetic diseases. Artificial abortion can be classified into two methods: surgical abortion and medical abortion.

*Chelsea B. Polis's research showed that most **induced abortions** in Malawi are performed under unsafe conditions, contributing to Malawi's high maternal mortality ratio.*

EXERCISES

Task 1: Vocabulary Application

Fill in the blanks with the words given below. Change the form where necessary.

> preventive; abuse; improve; prenatal; overlook; menarche; experience; detection; abortions; lifespans

1. The concept of _____ health care screening has been developed over the last 30 years through clinical trials of screening maneuvers, as well as a theoretical statistical literature.

2. Since medical problems can affect women and men differently, some serious medical issues may be _____ because symptoms in many women are not clear-cut.

3. Health care for women includes the entire spectrum of a woman's life. At each stage of a woman's life, it is very important to provide early _____ of medical problems, or to prevent them.

4. Self-care is anything we do to take care of our mental, emotional, and physical health. Self-care can _____ our mood and reduce anxiety, so it is always a good idea to take some time for yourself.

5. Our mental health can change during our lifetime. Women are known for putting others first and can _____ some mental health conditions at higher rates than men.

6. Urban women in age at _____ to a maximum of 15 years, rural women to 16 years of age the most.

7. The reason of most _____ is unwanted pregnancy.

8. Although most _____ tests simply confirm that a baby is healthy, it is important to prepare for other possibilities before giving birth.

9. As _____ lengthen, a person could still retire at 65 years old, but with a smaller annual benefit.

10. Alcohol and drug _____ among minors has long been a major problem for the

government there.

Task 2: Writing

For this part, you are allowed 30 minutes to write a composition on the topic of "The Harm of Early Life Adversity for Women". You should write at least 120 words, and base your composition on the outline below:

1) *What adverse outcomes does the early life adversity lead to among women?*

2) *How can we evaluate the early life adversity exposure in adult women?*

3) *What measures should we take to reduce the harm caused by early life adversity.*

Task 3: Oral Presentation

As we all know, health is important, but many women do not pay much attention to their health because they need to take care of many things about their families and work. Give them some advice about health and tell them the importance of women's health.

Learning Garden

Social Determinants for Child Obesity

According to social determinants of health (SDH) frameworks, child obesity is influenced by genetic, environmental and socio-cultural factors. Obesity is a complex multi-gene disease; in other words, genetic factors form the internal basis of obesity. Studies have found that parental weight can influence the occurrence of overweight and obesity in children through genetic factors, and children with both obese parents have a higher risk of obesity than those with neither obese parents. The obesity environment includes the change in dietary structure, such as high fat and sugar intake, decreased physical activity, increased sedentary time, and eating behaviors like skipping breakfast and consuming sugary drinks excessively. Additionally, frequent consumption of fast food is also a contributing factor. For example, parents driving their children to and from school has led to reduced energy expenditure and an increased risk of obesity. Social and economic status is another important factor that affects the occurrence and development of childhood obesity. In some developed countries, children with low socioeconomic status have higher obesity rates compared to those with high socioeconomic status; however, in China, the opposite trend can be observed. Particularly concerning is the influence of TV advertising on child obesity since most food advertisements on TV promote high-fat, high-sugar ,or high-salt foods. The amount of time children spend watching TV is positively correlated with the frequency of asking their parents to buy the food advertised on TV, which may contribute to the spread of obesity.

（范引光、杨淑娟）

Unit 7   Health Education

READING A

PREVIEW

In the field of public health, researchers and practitioners have examined three principal relationships between education and health. Firstly, health is a prerequisite for education: children who are hungry or hard of hearing, or children with chronic dental pain, for example, are **hampered** *in their learning. Secondly, health education occurs in schools and through various public health interventions; it is a central tool of public health. Thirdly, physical education in schools combines educating about the importance of physical activity for health with promoting such activity.*

Questions for Discussion

Q1: How does education affect health?
Q2: Why is health education important?

Text A

Health Education and Health Promotion

Health education is a part of health care that involves health-promoting behaviors. Since an individual's behavior can be the primary cause of a health problem, it can also be the main **solution**. Through health education, we help people understand how their behavior affects their health and encourage them to make their own choices for a healthy life without **coercion**. Health education aims to promote behavioral changes among individuals, groups, and larger populations by shifting people away from behaviors **perceived** as **detrimental** to their current and future health, towards those that are beneficial.

Health education covers the **continuum** from disease prevention and the promotion of **optimal** health to the detection, treatment, **rehabilitation**, and long-term care of illnesses. It includes infectious and chronic diseases as well as environmental concerns. Therefore, Health education is defined as "*any combination of learning experiences designed to facilitate voluntary actions conducive to health*".

In general, health education is the process by which individuals and groups learn to act in ways that facilitate the promotion, **maintenance**, or **restoration** of health. The *Alma-Ata Declaration*

(1978) emphasizes the need for individual and community involvement and offers a definition: *"a process designed to encourage people to want to be healthy, to know how to stay healthy, to do what they can individually and collectively to maintain health, and to seek help when needed"*.

Health Promotion

To achieve a state of complete physical, mental, and social well-being goes beyond the scope of health education or even the health sectors. In other words, health is not only the **responsibility** of health sector, but also of every sector **committed** to development. Thus, the concern for health beyond the health sector is a call for health promotion.

Health promotion is the process of enabling people to increase their control over and improve their health. It is a positive concept that emphasizes personal, social, political, and institutional resources as well as physical **capacities**. Health promotion is an umbrella term that includes disease prevention, health improvement, and enhancement of well-being.

Health promotion can be defined as *"a combination of educational and environmental supports for actions and living conditions that are conducive to health"*.

Health education is one of the most important **components** of health promotion. It is a means of promoting health. Health education primarily focuses on voluntary actions that individuals can take to improve their own health, as well as the health of their families and communities. Health promotion aims to take social and political actions to translate individual actions into health enhancement with necessary organizational, economic, and environmental support. In general, health promotion encompasses any combination of initiatives related to health education, economics, politics, spirituality or organization designed to bring about positive changes in attitudes, behaviors, society or environment that contribute to better population health.

Health Education in Disease Prevention

Disease prevention means interrupting or slowing the progression of a disease, with the aim of detecting and intervening in its risk factors. In health education, there are three different levels of disease prevention: primary, secondary, and tertiary health education.

1. Primary Health Education

It encompasses health education activities that are specifically designed to prevent illness or injury before the disease process begins, such as wearing seat belts, receiving **immunizations**, engaging in physical activities, and practicing breastfeeding.

2. Secondary Health Education

Once the disease has occurred, health education is important in slowing down the progression of the disease and preventing disability. For example, providing health education on adherence to treatment, educating patients to seek treatment, promoting breast cancer screening, conducting blood pressure examinations and **cholesterol** level screenings, as well as treating patients with **malaria**.

3. Tertiary Health Education

Health education programs specifically aimed at patients with **irreversible**, incurable, and chronic conditions can help with social and psychological adjustment, ultimately avoiding major disability and premature death. Examples include education after lung cancer surgery, and working with **diabetics** to ensure proper daily **injections**.

Health Education Settings

When considering the range of health education interventions, they are usually described in relation to different settings because interventions need to be planned in the light of the resources and organizational structures **peculiar** to each setting.

Health education is delivered in almost every conceivable setting-universities, schools, hospitals, pharmacies, grocery stores and shopping centers, recreational settings, community organizations, voluntary health agencies, worksites, churches, prisons, health maintenance organizations, and migrant labor camps. It is also delivered through mass media channels such as the Internet and in people's homes. Additionally, it is provided by health departments at all levels of government.

Thus, the main areas for health education and promotion activities are schools, worksites, healthcare settings, community settings, and special communities such as prisons and refugee settings. These settings differ in their organizational structure, the mission of the organization, and the centrality of the mission to health education. However, the process of health education is the same across settings, although there may be variations in content areas emphasized and target populations for health education.

1. Health Education Activities in School

School health education, as the name implies, primarily involves instructing school-age children about health and health-related behaviors. School children are a group of young people with similar backgrounds and environments. School-based health promotion is the most crucial approach for improving the well-being of children and adolescents.

2. Health Education Activities in Worksites

Health promotion encourages worksites to offer programs in worker safety and health, reduction of alcohol and smoking, education and control of blood pressure, and cholesterol. The majority of the activities reported at the worksites are focused on injury prevention, job hazards, and smoking control.

3. Health Education Activities in Health Care Setting

Health education for high-risk individuals, patients, their families, and the surrounding community, as well as in-service training for health care providers, is all part of health care today. It focuses on preventing and detecting diseases, helping people make decisions about genetic testing, and managing acute and chronic illnesses.

4. Health Education Activities in Homes

Health behavioral change interventions are delivered to people in their homes, both through traditional public health means, such as home visits, and through a variety of communication channels and media including the Internet, telephone, and mail.

Who is responsible for health education? While some are specially trained as specialists, it's crucial to recognize that all healthcare workers share the responsibility of enhancing people's health knowledge and skills. Failing to integrate health education into their daily work means they are not fulfilling their roles effectively. Thus, health education becomes the collective duty of everyone engaged in health and community development activities.

Challenges to the Process of Health Education

Good health education does not just happen; it requires much time, effort, practice, and on-the-job training to be successful. Even the most experienced health educators find program development challenging because no two days are the same in health education due to constant changes in settings, resources, and priority populations.

The process of health education is often challenging for several reasons: ①Health education is not considered as important during relatively healthy status as people are often more concerned about diseases. ②Changing health behavior is conditioned by factors such as social, psychological, economic, cultural aspects, accessibility and quality of services, and political environment which are difficult to deal with simultaneously. ③Many health professionals fail to recognize the value of health education.

Words and Expressions

hamper 阻碍，妨碍

*Studies show that cognitive development is severely **hampered** in malnourished children.*

solution （问题、困难等的）解决办法；（练习或竞赛的）解答，答案

*Engineers spend much time and energy developing brilliant **solutions**.*

coercion 强迫；胁迫

*It was vital that the elections should be free of **coercion** or intimidation.*

perceive 感知；认为；察觉到；注意到；意识到

*Stress is widely **perceived** as contributing to coronary heart disease.*

continuum （相邻两者相似但起首与末尾截然不同的）连续体

*These various complaints are part of a **continuum** of ill-health.*

optimal 最优的；最佳的

*According to the World Health Organization, the **optimal** birth interval is between two and three years.*

rehabilitation 康复；恢复；善后

*It is an important breakthrough for many people who require assistance with walking and **rehabilitation**.*

maintenance 维修；维护

*Careful **maintenance** can extend the life of your car.*

restoration （规章制度等的）恢复；修复

*The **restoration** to the castle took a year and cost a lot of money.*

responsibility 责任；负责

*The new position invested her with a good deal of **responsibility**.*

commit 承诺，保证（做某事、遵守协议或遵从安排等）

*China is **committed** to opening its doors and encouraging foreign investment as a basic* *long-term national strategy.*

capacity　容纳能力；领悟（或理解、办事）能力

*To make the computer work at full **capacity**, the programmer has to think like the machine.*

cholesterol　胆固醇

*Scientists have established a correlation between **cholesterol** levels and heart disease.*

malaria　疟疾

*One of the side effects may be to change the geographical distribution of parasitic diseases such as **malaria**.*

irreversible　不可逆转的；无法复原（或挽回）的；不能倒转的

*The renationalisation of policy making is splitting Europe and risks causing **irreversible** damage.*

diabetes　糖尿病

*People with high blood pressure are especially vulnerable to **diabetes**.*

injection　注射

*The reason why the **injection** needs repeating every year is that the virus changes.*

peculiar　特有的；奇怪的；怪异的；不寻常的；（某人、某地、某种情况等）特殊的

*Exceptional achievements carry their own **peculiar** risks.*

Language Points

primary health education　一级健康教育

At the primary level, we could educate people to practice some preventive behaviors such as having a balanced diet so that they can protect themselves from developing diseases in the future.

*In our community's latest initiative, **primary health education** focuses on teaching children the importance of handwashing, balanced diets, and regular physical activity to instill lifelong healthy habits.*

secondary health education　二级健康教育

At the secondary level, we could educate people to visit their local health center when they experience symptoms of illness, such as fever, so that they can receive early treatment for their health problems.

*To combat the spread of sexually transmitted infections among young adults, our public health agency has introduced a **secondary health education** series that includes confidential testing services, educational workshops, and digital resources aimed at promoting safe sexual practices.*

tertiary health education　三级健康教育

At the tertiary level, we could educate people to take their medication appropriately and find ways of working towards rehabilitation from significant illness or disability.

*Our hospital's **tertiary health education** program for diabetes patients includes personalized nutritional counseling and physical activity plans, alongside regular monitoring, and management sessions, to empower patients in managing their condition effectively.*

EXERCISES

Task 1: Vocabulary Application

Fill in the blanks with the words given below. Change the form where necessary.

> irreversible; capacity; detrimental; hamper; rehabilitation; restoration; responsibility; component; optimal; maintenance

1. China is trying to make _____ use of educational resources so that rural and underdeveloped areas will get more support.

2. She feels a strong sense of _____ towards her employees.

3. She argues that watching too much TV is _____ a child's intellectual and social development.

4. A complex engine has many separate _____ , each performing a different function.

5. The main issues are growth and the _____ of global demand.

6. She could suffer _____ brain damage if she is not treated within seven days.

7. The vehicle would not have the _____ to make the journey on one tank of fuel.

8. Lemons provide nutrients essential for your health and good _____ of your body.

9. The emergence of such problems seriously _____ the development of enterprises.

10. Medical treatment can be combined with _____ of local functions.

Task 2: Writing

For this part, you are allowed 30 minutes to write a composition on the topic: Education in Health. You should write at least 120 words, and base your composition on the outline below:

1) Education plays a crucial role in promoting health.

2) Health education scenarios exist in various aspects of everyday life.

3) Health education employs a variety of methods.

Task 3: Oral Presentation

The purpose of health education is to positively influence the health behavior of individuals and communities, as well as the living and working conditions that influence their health. Please try to describe how health behavior can be changed through health education.

READING B

PREVIEW

*Guizhou Province used to suffer from **endemic fluorosis** with the highest **prevalence**, the most patients, and the most severe degree of detriment. It was also known as the "miasmatic zone". Endemic fluorosis was also a factor restricting the economic development in Guizhou Province. Since the 1970s, Guizhou Province has commenced the promotion of **retrofitted** stoves. However, minimal effect was observed. From 2004 to 2010, the Guizhou Provincial Government* *extensively promoted prevention and control activities regarding retrofitted stoves. In addition, large-scale health education and health promotion practices were implemented. By 2010, a total of 3,986,500 retrofitted stoves had been installed in the province, and the utilization rate of retrofitted stoves had reached 99.34%. These outcomes took the pioneering lead in achieving full coverage of strategies for preventing and controlling endemic fluorosis throughout the country, making a historic breakthrough in disease control activities. Up to 2019, endemic fluorosis has been basically eliminated in 37 disease-related regions (counties) in Guizhou Province.*

Questions for Discussion

Q1: What is the significance of health education in rural areas of China?

Q2: Have you ever received health education in your life? If so, what kind of health education have you received?

Text B

Overcome Endemic Fluorosis Through Health Education and Retrofitted Stoves Activities in Guizhou Province

Zhijin County, located in Bijie District of Guizhou Province, was an **impoverished** ethnic minority county that received support from the national government. Lotus Village is located 10 kilometers away from Zhijin County. Since the 1970s, the village has been **stricken** with a strange disease, where people with **stooped** backs could be seen everywhere. Additionally, these people had yellow and black teeth as well as X-shaped (knock knees) or O-shaped (bow legs) legs, and their arms could only be bent but not stretched. Moreover, barely villagers could reach up to 1.7 meters tall, and most of them were very **skinny**. People in that village rarely lived to 70 years old, and usually died before 50 or 60 years old.

What on earth was this strange disease? After a thorough **investigation**, it turned out that the disease suffered by these villagers was **endemic fluorosis**. In 1979, the Guizhou Provincial Epidemic Prevention Station and the Institute of Geochemistry of the Chinese Academy of Sciences conducted a survey in the Lotus Village. Surprisingly, the **prevalence** of dental fluorosis among people over 8 years old was 100%, and the prevalence of **skeletal** fluorosis was as high as 77.6%. Guizhou Province was a severely affected area by endemic fluorosis as a result of coal **combustion**. There were approximately 10 million dental fluorosis patients and 1 million skeletal fluorosis patients in the province. Up to about 15 million people were affected by endemic fluorosis, accounting for half the population of the national cases. The causes for these phenomena were included in the following aspects:

(1) Rural residents in Guizhou Province used open stoves without **chimneys** for heating, and they had the habit of burning coal mixed with clay. Although the **fluorine** content in coal was within the normal range, the fluorine content in clay far **exceeded** the normal value. Under such long-term combustion, the fluorine **concentration** in the air often exceeds the standard.

(2) It was common for residents in rural Guizhou to warm themselves in front of a fire, roast corn and chili on the house, because of the cold and **humid** weather in the southwest mountain area of China. After the autumn harvest, various kinds of crops must be dried up for storage purposes. The villagers often used open **stoves** without chimneys to bake crops. However, crops such as corn and chili had a strong capability to absorb fluorine. After roasting, the fluorine content of these crops could exceed the national standard by dozens or even hundreds of times.

(3) In the local area, villagers barely **rinsed** the roasted crops such as corn and chili prior to cooking. They usually cooked and ate these crops directly after some rough processing.

In short, the combination of the natural environment and habitual behavior made people exposed to a high fluoride environment for a long time, which eventually made Guizhou Province a severely affected area of endemic fluorosis. As a result, this led to a vicious circle of poverty-induced disease and disease-induced poverty, which severely constrained socio-economic development.

In order to eradicate endemic fluorosis, the government has tried to provide free medical services, but the effect was not satisfactory. This is because there was no effective treatment for endemic fluorosis. Under this circumstance, the main work should be focused on disease prevention. The results of the epidemiological survey showed that the main cause of endemic fluorosis in Guizhou is the above-mentioned habitual behaviors. To prevent endemic fluorosis, the simplest and most important strategy is to promote utilization of chimneys discharging smoke from the house, which could effectively prevent people and food from being directly exposed to high fluoride environments. Therefore, the program of **retrofitting** stoves commenced in the 1970s. Guizhou Province established a province-wide prevention and control plan for endemic fluorosis. However, the seemingly simple "stove revolution" encountered numerous obstacles in its implementation.

On the one hand, there were three million stoves in Guizhou Province that required to be retrofitted, but the annual government investment funds were limited. It took 150-170 yuan to retrofit a stove. Although the government invested proportionally, and only 20 yuan was required to be paid per household, many villagers still could not afford it, resulting in a slow process of retrofitting stoves. Moreover, the chimneys of retrofitted stoves needed to be replaced every one or two years,, and a chimney would cost 100 yuan. Many farmers were also reluctant to pay for it. Therefore, after the chimney was broken, the retrofitted stoves functioned like an open stove. On the other hand, even in the small-scale pilot programs, retrofitted stoves did not show their effectiveness. Because in the view of many villagers, the retrofitted stoves could not hold the pots and could only be used for heating. As for cooking pig feed and roasting crops, open stoves seemed to be a better choice for them. In addition, after using the retrofitted stoves, although the fluorine concentration decreased significantly indoors, it also lowered the efficiency of drying crops and **prolonged** the time required for drying. Therefore, the degree of fluorine contamination in foods such as corn and chili has not been decreased. Finally, the "stove revolution" could not effectively prevent and control endemic fluorosis.

Since there was no effective treatment for endemic fluorosis, the prevention and control of endemic fluorosis turned out to be essential. However, through incessant exploration by the prevention and control team, they have found that the program of retrofitting stoves alone is ineffective. In order to make the villagers aware of the significance of preventing and controlling endemic fluorosis, health education and health promotion practices for the public were the top priority. Villagers should have a comprehensive understanding of the **hazards** of endemic fluorosis, the benefits of retrofitted stoves, as well as the significance of modifying unhealthy behaviors. It was vital to inform them of both benefits and harms, so that they could consciously fight against endemic fluorosis.

In the early days after the founding of the People's Republic of China, Guizhou Province had 37 districts (counties) endemic to fluorosis, with a population of approximately 15 million. Among them, there were nearly 11 million patients suffering from dental fluorosis and skeletal fluorosis. Since the 1970s, Guizhou has been implementing measures to retrofit stoves in districts where endemic fluorosis was prevalent. However, minimal effect was observed. After the mid-1990s, a prevention and control team conducted research on health education and behavioral intervention for endemic fluorosis in Democracy Township, Longli County, Qiannan Buyi and Miao Autonomous Prefecture, Guizhou Province. The awareness rate of knowledge about endemic fluorosis prevention and control had risen from 2% to 80% in this area two years later. Approximately 70% of the population had **fostered** the habit of not using open stoves to roast food such as corn and chili, and rinsing the food prior to cooking. Due to effective measures for prevention and control of endemic fluorosis in this region, the indoor air fluoride concentration was within the national standard, and the urine fluoride level of children aged 8 to 12 also tended to be normal.

In the large-scale endemic fluorosis prevention and control activities, Guizhou Province adopted a combination of interpersonal communication and mass communication to carry out health education activities in the following four aspects:

First of all, it was recommended to repeatedly broadcast public service announcements on the hazards of endemic fluorosis and its prevention and control through radio, newspapers, television, and other mass media. Then targeted core information and easy-to-understand knowledge of endemic fluorosis prevention and control could be spread through wall slogans, spray paintings, and rural broadcasting, which could deepen the public's awareness of endemic fluorosis, and thus formed a conscious awareness of endemic fluorosis prevention and control.

Secondly, village cadres and health prevention and control staff who have been trained in the knowledge related to endemic fluorosis were organized to visit the disease areas, convene village committees to disseminate the core knowledge of endemic fluorosis, communicate with the public repeatedly to convince them to accept the retrofitted stoves. In addition, in-depth education should be implemented from the family perspective, by conducting face-to-face prevention and control education, so that the knowledge would be firmly "remembered".

Thirdly, on market days, health staff would carefully explain the severity of endemic fluorosis to the human body and how to prevent and control it to passers-by through the distribution of leaflets and propaganda materials, on-site consultation, and other forms in order to **expand** the scope of health education.

Fourthly, health education was implemented in schools. Health education classes were held for the young generation in the disease area to inculcate new concepts on the prevention and control of endemic fluorosis; the prevention and control of fluorosis were publicized on special columns and blackboards; students were organized to go into farming households and carry out practical activities of "small hands holding big hands", so that children could convince their parents and adults to deepen their understanding of the hazards of endemic fluorosis as well as its prevention and control.

Up to 2010, Guizhou Province had retrofitted stoves in a total of 3,986,500 households, with the utilization rate of retrofitted stoves reaching as high as 99.34%, taking the pioneering lead in achieving full coverage of endemic fluorosis prevention and control strategies throughout the country. Up to 2019, endemic fluorosis has been basically eliminated in Guizhou Province. Moreover, the retrofitted stoves have significantly reduced the pollution from coal combustion, reduced the use of non-renewable energy, and to a certain extent improved environmental health and protected the ecological environment in the disease areas. The prevention and control of endemic fluorosis in Guizhou Province have formed a comprehensive prevention strategy combining health education, health promotion, and stove conversion. Because the strategy was advanced and maneuverable, it has been promoted and applied in other endemic fluorosis areas nationwide.

Words and Expressions

impoverished　贫困的, 赤贫的;(品质)恶化的
*He warned that the breakdown of the family unit would lead to an **impoverished** society.*

stricken　受灾的, 患病的, 受困扰的
*Whole villages were **stricken** with the disease.*

stooped　弓背站立(或行走)的;驼背的, 曲背的
*Postmenopausal osteoporosis is common and is associated with **stooped** posture, loss of height, back pain, and fractures.*

investigation　调查, 科学研究
*Epidemiological **investigations** of outbreaks of infectious disease must be carried out rapidly but must be methodologically sound.*

endemic　地方性的
*Keshan disease is an **endemic** cardiomyopathy in humans.*

fluorosis　(慢性)氟中毒
*High levels of fluoride from food and contaminated groundwater are putting many people in India at risk of **fluorosis**, an underappreciated and sometimes debilitating disease.*

prevalence　流行, 盛行
*The **prevalence** of several silkworm diseases has led to a decline in silk products.*

skeletal　骨骼的
***Skeletal** muscle is the protein reservoir of our body and an important regulator of glucose and lipid homeostasis.*

combustion　燃烧;(化学)氧化,(化学)燃烧;骚动
*The energy is released by **combustion** on the application of a match.*

chimney　烟囱, 烟道

*Puffs of white smoke came from the **chimney**.*

fluorine　氟

*The abundance of **fluorine** in the environment as well as in drinking water sources are the major contributors to fluorosis.*

exceed　超过, 超出; 超越(限制)

*Your intake of alcohol should not **exceed** two units per day.*

concentration　浓度, 含量

*The **concentration** of oxygen dissolved in tissues at the time of irradiation is an influence factor of radiotherapy.*

humid　潮湿的, 湿热的

*These plants love warm, **humid** atmospheres.*

stove　(取暖或烹饪用的)炉子, 火炉; 厨灶, 炉头; 窑

*She put a pan of water on the **stove**.*

rinse　冲洗, 漱

*All subjects received scaling and polishing to remove plaque, extrinsic stain, and calculus and then **rinsed** with their allocated mouth rinse.*

retrofit　改造, 改进

*This sample model is designed to **retrofit** existing microscopic crowd models to perform the assessments of occupant exposure.*

prolong　延长, 拉长

*Various types of formulations have been widely used to **prolong** the residence time of the dosage form at the site of application.*

hazard　危险, 危害; (不可避免的)风险

*The recent outbreaks of cholera are a timely reminder that this disease is still a serious health **hazard**.*

foster　养成, 培养, 促进

*We conducted this activity to educate and motivate the youth to **foster** healthy sleep habits.*

expand　扩大, 增大, 放大

*Stricture prevention is necessary to allow for endoscopic therapy to **expand**.*

Language Points

dental fluorosis　氟斑牙

Dental fluorosis, also called mottling of tooth enamel, is a developmental disturbance of dental enamel caused by excessive exposure to high concentrations of fluoride during tooth development.

*Fluoridated water is, directly or indirectly, responsible for 40% of **dental fluorosis**, through water intake or children's formula and food prepared with drinking water.*

skeletal fluorosis　氟骨症

Skeletal fluorosis is a pathophysiological condition caused by high levels of fluoride accumulation in bones and joints via inhalation or ingestion over a chronic period.

*The major symptoms associated with the **skeletal fluorosis** are chronic joint pain, stiffness* *of joint, sporadic pain, calcification of ligaments and osteosclerosis.*

vicious circle　恶性循环

Vicious circle refers to complex chains of events that reinforce themselves through a feedback loop.

*This **vicious circle** implies that stress can increase magnesium loss, causing a deficiency; in turn, magnesium deficiency can enhance the body's susceptibility to stress.*

top priority　最优先的, 当务之急

The thing that is most important.

*The **top priority** is building a better system for tobacco-cessation counseling.*

interpersonal communication　人际传播

Interpersonal communication is the process of exchange of information, ideas, and feelings between two or more people through verbal or non-verbal methods.

***Interpersonal communication** is born through the combination of verbal, nonverbal and paraverbal forms.*

mass communication　大众传播

Mass communication is the process of imparting and exchanging information through mass media to large segments of the population.

***Mass communication** techniques are currently limited in nursing; however, they are predicted to hold great promise in the future.*

EXERCISES

Task 1: Vocabulary Application

Fill in the blanks with the words given below. Change the form where necessary.

> **stooped; investigation; endemic; skeletal; rinse; retrofit; prolong; foster; expand; concentration**

1. Hepatitis B is _____ in China and other parts of Asia.

2. One important difference between a chimpanzee and human, is their _____ muscle structure.

3. In order to _____ healthy dietary and physical activity habits among middle aged African Americans, we have carried out this health education and health promotion activity.

4. The effect of physiotherapy on _____ posture in Parkinson's disease patients remains to be clarified.

5. Fluorine may pose possible health risks to children in high fluorine _____ areas.

6. Excluding subjects from research for the only reason of belonging to a vulnerable group is unethical and will bias the results of the _____ .

7. Hydrogen peroxide at the recommended oral _____ concentrations of 1.5% and 3.0% was minimally effective as a viricidal agent after contact times as long as 30 seconds.

8. Many psychotropic medications may further _____ this interval.

9. Transitional age _____ youth benefit from policies promoting a developmentally

appropriate, comprehensive, and integrated transition system of care.

10. Pharmaceutical companies have a moral obligation to _____ access to investigational drugs to patients outside the clinical trial.

Task 2: Writing

For this part, you are allowed 30 minutes to write a composition on the topic: Health education in epidemic prevention and control. You should write at least 120 words, and base your composition on the outline below:

1) The significance of raising public awareness in terms of epidemic prevention and control.

2) What factors should be taken into consideration when addressing health education issues in case-specific regions (ethnic minorities etc.)?

3) What methodologies should we adopt to implement appropriate health education activities? Please also outline all relevant perspectives and provide an example of their corresponding detailed approaches.

Task 3: Oral Presentation

Health education strives to improve people's health awareness and cultivate skills that will assist them in maintaining their health. Health education is critical for improving the overall health of different communities and people. It will also contribute to the overall health of the nation. You may also say that the economy of a country is directly proportional to health education.

Please describe how health education imposes a positive effect from the perspective of individuals, communities, and nations. From the view of young generation, please propose some innovative approaches to raise public awareness regarding epidemic prevention and control (Hint: new media, technologies, and people's daily behavior).

Learning Garden

Ottawa Charter for Health Promotion

The Ottawa Charter for Health Promotion is the name of an international agreement signed at the First International Conference on Health Promotion, organized by the World Health Organization (WHO) and held in Ottawa, Canada, in November 1986. It launched a series of actions among international organizations, national governments and local communities to achieve the goal of "Health For All" by the year 2000 and beyond through better health promotion.

Five action areas for health promotion were identified in the charter:

1. Building healthy public policy
2. Creating supportive environments
3. Strengthening community action
4. Developing personal skills
5. Re-orienting health care services toward prevention of illness and promotion of health

（范颂、卢雍）

Unit 8   Systems Epidemiology

READING A

PREVIEW

In the last century, epidemiologists predominantly focused on identifying disease risk factors using "black box" epidemiology, which primarily aimed to uncover simple and straightforward associations between exposures and diseases. While this approach yielded valuable insights, it had significant limitations. Critics argued that this approach merely generated a list of risk factors without shedding light on a biological and medical foundation. In addition, this approach failed to reveal intrinsic relationships among risk factors, which often interact with one another forming complex networks. Consequently, associations identified using the "black box" approach in one study frequently contradicted those in another. In the absence of a more advanced theory and approach, our ability to effectively predict intervention effects in the field of public health remains constrained.

Questions for Discussion

Q1: What challenges did traditional epidemiology, also known as "black box epidemiology", encounter?

Q2: What potential strategies can be employed to address these challenges?

Text A

Systems Theory in Disease Modelling and Application in Infectious Disease

Opening the "black box" can be achieved through two primary approaches: the first involves leveraging established methods, such as medication analysis and causal inference, to partially unveil it. Alternatively, a systems-based strategy can be employed. While the former is more mature for mathematical simplification, the latter holds greater promise, as it aligns with the complex nature of the etiology of diseases, which result from the intricate interactions of numerous factors.

The foundational theory underlying the modeling of disease occurrence and progression from a systems perspective draws from Ludwig Von Bertalanffy's *General System Theory*, proposed in 1940. Bertalanffy's assertion that "the whole is more than the sum of its parts", represents a distinct departure from **reductionism**. He further emphasized that the application of system analysis to biological system should be one of the central goals of general system theory.

While the general system theory provides the theoretical foundation, the remarkable advancements in molecular biology technology have offered the practical means to apply these concepts. Key technological breakthroughs, such as the discovery of the double helix structure of DNA by James Watson and Francis Crick in 1953 (Nobel Prize in 1962) and the development of the rapid DNA and protein sequencing technology by Frederick Sanger in 1977 (Nobel Prize 1980), have enabled the profiling of DNA, RNA, and protein sequences across various biological layers of the human body. This groundwork laid the essential foundation for **systems biology**, an **interdisciplinary** endeavor that integrates molecular, cellular, tissue, organ, and organism-level functions into computational models for identifying biological pathways and networks. In 2002, the journal *NATURE* published a special issue highlighting systems biology, introducing topics like the genomic regulatory network for development and modelling the heart from genes to cells to the whole organ. In comparison to systems biology, **systems medicine**, also known as network medicine, focuses specifically on diseases and explores not only biological networks but also disease networks.

Compared with systems biology and systems medicine, **systems epidemiology** introduces an additional layer of consideration, accounting for **antecedents** that may contribute to disease progression in populations. In 2014, Dammann and colleagues summarized the concept of systems epidemiology as an epidemiologic approach that encompasses (i) systems-level **exposure** measurements (e.g., omics) at multiple levels (e.g.,**sociodemographic**, clinical, biological); (ii) network analyses of **interrelationships** among risk factors and (iii) computational simulation of risk scenarios in parallel to **data-driven** biostatistical risk modelling. Over the past decades, systems epidemiology has seen development primarily in terms of design and methodology. The field encourages the creation of computational simulation models that integrate information on disease **etiology**, pathogenetic data, and insights from experts from diverse **disciplines**. This systems-based approach, considering multiple levels of causation, allows epidemiologists to gain a more comprehensive understanding of contributors and their interactions in the development of various diseases. Such knowledge contributes to improving **syndromic surveillance** methods in public health research and practice.

The need for a systems epidemiology approach in infectious disease research was first underscored in the context of tuberculosis (TB). TB, caused by *Mycobacterium tuberculosis*, primarily affects the lungs and presents a global health challenge. Approximately one-quarter of the world's population is estimated to be latently infected with TB bacteria according to the World Health Organization. In 2020, TB claimed 1.5 million lives, ranking as the 13th leading cause of death and the second leading infectious killer after COVID-19, surpassing HIV/AIDS. The outcome of TB infection vary significantly, ranging from complete bacterial clearance by the host's **innate immunity**, to typical **pulmonary** disease, **disseminated** TB, or even death. While around 90% of infected individuals remain in a latent state, 5%-10% eventually develop active TB during their lifetime. The intricate interplay between the pathogen and the host immune system largely determines individual outcomes. To effectively combat TB globally, effective tools for diagnostics, **antibiotics** and vaccines are imperative. Several breakthroughs have been made, such as the identification of an **interferon**-inducible **neutrophil**-driven blood transcriptional signature, enabling the identification of infected individuals at higher risk of progressing to active TB. Additionally, antibiotics, including **streptomycin** (developed in 1943), **ethambutol** (developed in 1960s) and a few other anti-TB drugs, have been developed, though long-term administration has led to drug resistance. The Bacille Calmette-Guérin (BCG) vaccine, while not without limitations, effectively protects children against TB **meningitis**, the most severe form of TB infection.

Despite the remarkable progress in TB research over the past decade, significant knowledge gaps persist in understanding the basic biology of *Mycobacterium tuberculosis* and its **crosstalks** with the human host. A systems-based approach is increasingly recognized as essential for the development of new diagnostics, drugs, and vaccines against TB. The chronic and complex nature of TB, characterized by the interplay between the pathogen and the host immune system, **latency**, mycobacterial cell wall complexity, antimicrobial persistence, and the vaccine's effectiveness, necessitates a systems-oriented understanding of TB infection and progression.

Consequently, two systems biology **initiatives**, the TB Systems Biology Program and SysteMTb, were launched to investigate TB. These initiatives are funded by the National Institutes of Health/National Institute of Allergy and Infectious Diseases (NIH/NIAID) and the European Union (EU), respectively. They encourage research that applies high-throughput technologies and computational modeling to integrate and interpret complex biological data. Genomics, transcriptomics, regulatomics, proteomics and metabolomics have all gained **momentum** in TB research.

However, systems biology alone is insufficient to address all aspects of infectious diseases like TB. Host and pathogen diversity, changes in human **demography**, socioeconomic and environmental factors, should also be taken into consideration. In England and Wales, a decline in TB mortality had already commenced long before the identification of TB's causative agent by Robert Koch in 1890 and the introduction of the first anti-TB drug streptomycin in 1943, as well as the BCG vaccination in 1950. This trend suggests that improvements in living conditions, nutrition and sanitation likely played a pivotal role in diminishing the TB epidemic. Consequently, questions arise regarding the specific contributions of anti-TB treatment and BCG vaccination to the overall reduction of TB in Europe. Moreover, the interplay between human host genetic diversity and TB strain diversity significantly influences susceptibility to TB, the process of immune recognition, and virulence. This complex scenario necessitates an enhanced understanding of the multifaceted interactions among numerous factors, encompassing elements of systems biology, epidemiology, sociology, the evolutionary history of hosts and pathogens, as well as ecology. This integrated approach collectively encompasses both the physical and social environments and is encapsulated as "systems epidemiology".

Words and Expressions

reductionism　简化论

*Algorithmism asserts that phenomena and process of biosis are computable, and this assertion has gone on with **reductionism**.*

systems　系统

***Systems** biology is the computational and mathematical analysis and modeling of complex biological systems.*

antecedent　先例，前因

*This study reveals the association between **antecedent** blood pressure, hypertension-mediated organ damage and cardiovascular outcome.*

exposure　暴露

*This narrative review summarizes recently published epidemiological and in vivo experimental studies on **exposure** to environmental chemicals and their potential role in the development of type 1 diabetes mellitus (T1DM).*

sociodemographic　社会人口的

*Clinical and **sociodemographic** characteristics were compared between the groups.*

interrelationship　相互关系

*In this study, we seek to explore the set of **interrelationship**s between all of the variables of sport, social capital, health, and subjective well-being.*

data-driven　数据驱动

***Data-driven** science removes the assumption that the scientist has adequate biologic insight to generate the best specific, testable hypotheses.*

discipline　学科

*The core public health **disciplines** include biostatistics, epidemiology, health policy and management, social and behavioral sciences, and environmental health sciences.*

mycobacterium　分枝杆菌；分枝杆菌属

***Mycobacterium** avium is a bloodstream infection caused by a bacterium related to tuberculosis.*

innate　先天的；固有的；与生俱来的

*However, the molecular mechanism for **innate** immune recognition was unclear.*

immunity　免疫；免疫力

*The vaccine provides longer **immunity** against flu.*

pulmonary　肺的，肺部的

***Pulmonary** vessels include the **pulmonary** artery and its branches, and the veins that drain the lung capillaries.*

disseminated　弥散的，播散的

*No serum factor has been identified that can detect already **disseminated** breast cancer.*

antibiotics　抗生素

***Antibiotics** are medicines that fight bacterial infections in people and animals.*

interferon 干扰素

*Other T cells produce chemicals called lymphokines (such as **interferon**s and interleukins) that have a toxic effect upon cells or bacteria.*

neutrophil 中性粒细胞

*By slowing down the movement of **neutrophil**s, it prevents the cells from congregating in the lung area, thus relieving congestion.*

streptomycin 链霉素

*The main drug-resistant strain was **streptomycin**-resistant.*

ethambutol 乙胺丁醇

*This study seeks to comprehend the molecular mechanisms and expedited the identification of **ethambutol**-resistant Mycobacterium tuberculosis.*

meningitis 脑膜炎

*Meningitis is a disease caused by the inflammation of the protective membranes covering the brain and spinal cord known as the **meninges**.*

consensus （意见等）一致

*However, no **consensus** with regard to surgical options and resection margins as been reached so far.*

crosstalks 相互影响，串话

*Biological **crosstalks** refers to instances in which one or more components of one signal transduction pathway affects another.*

latency 潜伏期

*Infection **latency** refers to the period during which a pathogen remains dormant within a host before becoming active and causing symptoms.*

initiative 倡议

*Supplementation to prevent iron deficiency without anemia may be a community-based **initiative**.*

momentum 动力

*This IDC Perspective provides a step-by-step guide for CIOs and digital transformation leaders who want to foster continued **momentum** as they move from COVID-19 response to post-COVID-19 transformation.*

demography 人口统计学

*We can move from questions about **demography** and ask questions about human health.*

Language Points

Systems Epidemiology 系统流行病学

Systems epidemiology is an emerging field of epidemiology that integrates extensive medical data with systems biology. It investigates statistical models of disease risk, conducts future risk simulations, and predicts disease outcomes using data spanning molecular, cellular, population, social, and ecological levels. This term should be distinuighsed from related fields, such as systems biology (系统生物学) and systems medicine (系统医学).

The chronic nature of tuberculosis (TB), arising from intricate interactions between the host's immune system and the pathogen, necessitates the application of **systems epidemiology** *approaches to enhance diagnostics, antibiotics and vaccines.*

Black Box Epidemiology　黑匣流行病学

Black box epidemiology pertains to the utilization of observational epidemiological techniques and inference for deducing cause-effect relationships between risk factors and disease outcomes. This is done without the requirement of a comprehensive understanding or an attempt to elucidate intricate causal mechanisms or the specific disease's pathogenesis under investigation.

Black box epidemiology, as exemplified in John Snow's study of cholera in 1850s London, focuses on identifying associations between risk factors and disease outcomes without delving into the underlying causal mechanisms.

General Systems Theory　一般系统论

General systems theory is an interdisciplinary conceptual framework that centers on comprehending the entirety, patterns, relationship, hierarchical structures, integration, and organization of phenomena. Its purpose is to transcend the reductionist (简化的) and mechanistic (机械的) traditions in science, harmonizing fragmented approaches and diverse classes of phenomena investigated by modern science into a coherent and unified whole.

In the framework of **general systems theory,** *an entity or phenomenon is considered holistically as a collection of interacting elements, constituting a system. The overarching objective of general systems theory is to discern and comprehend the principles that are universally applicable to all systems. The influence of each element within a system is contingent upon the functions performed by other elements in that system, and the organization emerges from the interactions among these elements.*

EXERCISES

Task 1: Vocabulary Application
Fill in the blanks with the words given below. Change the form where necessary.

> **exposure; systems; sociodemographic; data-driven; antecedent; crosstalk; latency; initiative; discipline; interrelationship**

1. There are two types of methods for analyzing functional magnetic resonance imaging data: _____ methods and model-drive methods.

2. The _____ of public health seeks to promote and protect the health of people and their communities.

3. In biology, _____ between signaling pathways is a common phenomenon where different cellular communication systems interact, often influencing the cell's response to

various stimuli.

4. Prolonged _____ to harmful environmental pollutants can significantly impact human health, leading to various respiratory and cardiovascular conditions.

5. Clinical and _____ characteristics were compared between the groups.

6. The Precision Medicine _____, launched by the government, aims to tailor medical treatments to individual patients by considering their unique genetic and molecular profiles.

7. _____ epidemiology, with its focus on the interplay of various factors at molecular, population, and ecological levels, is crucial for comprehending and managing complex disease dynamics, such as infectious disease outbreaks.

8. The study sought to identify the _____ factors that contributed to the recent surge in urban population growth.

9. It uses this to interpret the _____ of the patterns and draw conclusions that allow us to identify people and places.

10. At the beginning of a COVID-19 infection, there is a period of time known as the exposed or _____ period, before an infected person is capable of transmitting the infection to another person.

Task 2: Writing

For this part, you are allowed 30 minutes to write a composition on the topic: Systems Epidemiology. You should write at least 120 words, and base your composition on the outline below:

1) Limitations of "black box epidemiology".

2) Potential ways of revolving those limitations.

3) Difference between the "black box epidemiology" and "systems epidemiology" approaches.

4) Difference between systems epidemiology, systems biology, and systems medicine.

Task 3: Oral Presentation

Systems epidemiology has been used in research of infectious diseases such as influenza, Zika, tuberculosis and COVID-19, etc. Please provide an example of how scientists apply systems epidemiology to study and contain a specific infectious disease.

READING B

PREVIEW

Recent advancements in "omics" "biosensor" and "imaging" technologies have empowered epidemiologists to introduce innovative biomarkers at various levels in human observational reseach. This has the potential to shift the traditional research paradigm away from the black-box strategy towards a systems approach, enabling a deeper understanding of disease etiology beyond mere associations. This new model encompasses a comprehensive array of information-including genetic predisposition (genome), epigenetic alterations (epigenome), gene expression (transcriptome), protein profiles (proteome), metabolites (metabolome), gut microbiota composition (microbiome), and exposure data (exposome). These components are integrated into population-based studies, enriching our insights into the biological mechanisms and the intricate interplay between individuals and their environment, elucidating the pathophysiology of diseases in human populations.

Questions for Discussion

Q1: What do you consider the most essential elements in conducting a systems epidemiology study of a specific disease?

Q2: Can you provide examples of chronic disease studies that have effectively applied systems epidemiology principles?

Text B

Advances in Systems Epidemiology for Non-Communicable Diseases

Systems epidemiology has been used in studies of non-communicable diseases, such as Type II Diabetes, cardiovascular disease and cancer. It has also informed causality in the field of nutritional epidemiology, for example, exploring coffee as a potential therapy for health effects. A notable initial success has been achieved in cancer research.

In cancer epidemiology over the past decades, prospective studies have largely retained their design, centering on gene-environment interactions. These studies make extensive use of biobank resources, emphasizing DNA analyses, and employ diagnosed cancers as primary outcomes. Within this framework, exposure data from questionnaires, biomarkers, and single nucleotide polymorphisms are considered as variables, assessed for associations with reported cancer cases. Despite the wealth of data collected, elements such as the transcriptome, proteome, and other molecular intricacies remain enigmatic "black boxes." **Up-to-date** technologies have opened new horizons for interactive studies, offering opportunities to integrate genetic predisposition (DNA-**genome**), gene expression (**transcriptome**), protein profiles (**proteome**), and metabolites (**metabolome**) with lifestyle information collected via questionnaires. This comprehensive approach extends our capacity to investigate gene variants, gene expression and modifications, proteins, and signaling and metabolic pathways, enhancing the understanding of disease etiology and progression.

Towards this end, the Cancer Genome Atlas (TCGA) was initiated in 2006 as an international **landmark** program dedicated to the comprehensive molecular characterization of over 20,000 **primary** cancer cases, complemented by paried normal samples covering 33 different types of cancers. The primary mission of TCGA was to illuminate the diverse facets of cancer hallmarks by discerning commonalities and disparities in genomic and cellular **alterations**. The program encouraged **multidisciplinary** collaboration across countries and time zones, involving researches such as mathematicians, bioinformaticians, statisticians, biologists, epidemiologists and clinicians among others. By the end of 2018, TCGA had generated over 2.5 **petabytes** of data encompassing genomic (exome sequencing, copy number and chromosomal **aneuploidy**), epigenomic (DNA methylation), transcriptomic (mRNA and miRNA sequencing), and proteomic (a cancer-relevant set of proteins and **phosphoproteins**) profiles for around 10,000 tumor specimens.

Leveraging this extensive dataset, researchers harnessed the power of machine learning, sometimes referred to as Artificial Intelligence, to perform molecular classifications of tumors. This process involved a comparative analysis of the molecular **taxonomy** with the conventional organ-tissue-**histology**-based **pathology** classification; to extract "stemness" features from normal **embryonic** cells and their **progenitors**; and to identify important biological networks that can contribute to potential drug targets for anti-cancer therapies. Computer models were trained to identify similar features across cancer cells originating from over thirty tumor types. These data-driven investigations led to several noteworthy findings: (I) The cell-of-origin has a strong influence on DNA methylation pattern, though it does not entirely determine tumor classification; (II) Identification of novel molecular taxonomies that exhibit significant divergence from the conventional organ-tissue-histology-based pathology classification. Such findings are particularly valuable, as this new subclassification system has the potential to enhance the management of 1%-3% of newly diagnosed cancer patients with cancer of unknown primary (CUP); (III) Immune features derived from mRNA profiling and copy-number aberrations are pivotal in defining the most heterogeneous tumor groups. This applies even to tumors with shared characteristics in terms of tumor type, organ system, and histopathology; (IV) Cancer **abuses** cellular mechanisms that are active in normal development for its oncogenic progression and formation of **metastases** , which can be used to **stratify** cancer patients for immunotherapies with stem cells-based vaccines; (V) Several tumors, for example, **stromal** and **mesenchymal** tumors are commonly enriched for gene programs representing PD1, CTLA4, and GP2-T cell or B cell activation, indicating that new therapies targeting such specific immune pathways may be appropriate.

In sum, the **integrative** study design and analysis of TCGA within the framework of systems epidemiology has led to valuable insights into cancer subgroups, shedding light on stem-cell-like features associated with **oncogenic dedifferentiation**. This profound comprehension of cancer's etiology and classification, in comparison to traditional epidemiology, enables and promotes breakthroughs in cancer diagnosis, treatment and prevention.

Recent advancements have ushered in a new research discipline within epidemiology, known as systems epidemiology, offering the potential to position epidemiology at the forefront of technological and scientific advancements. This shift could fundamentally transform the **paradigm** of chronic non-communicable disease epidemiology. However, the journey ahead is not without **momentous** challenges. Central to this endeavor is the role of computational modeling, which serves as a cornerstone for comprehending the emergence and progression of diseases. Computational simulations yield valuable insights into the intricate interplay of risk factors across various levels, thereby elucidating the complex processes underlying human diseases. Nonetheless, meticulously **simulating** multi-level research designs remains a formidable task. The ongoing challenge lies in the development and execution of network analyses to dissect interactions within the layers of the system.

Another formidable challenge confronting systems epidemiology pertains to the **standardization** and **unification** of multi-omics data, including biomarkers. Leveraging advanced computational modeling techniques necessitates the creation of an integrated platform and dataset capable of amalgamating highly dynamic data parameters. It is imperative to evaluate the relationship between omics-level phenotypes and other phenotypes, with a specific focus on dynamic exposure factors. This integration must seamlessly bridge the gap between **experimental** data and **theoretical** modeling. The Cancer Genome Atlas (TCGA) program stands as a notable exemplar of systems epidemiological research in our field.

Most importantly, the integration of systems biology and systems epidemiology poses a significant question. The aspiration is to swiftly apply computational models of the pathogenic mechanisms from systems biology to computational etiology models that simulate the onset of human diseases. However, the key to this integration rests in interdisciplinary **cooperation**. Only through strengthened cooperation among systems biologists, epidemiologists, and computer scientists can we harmoniously meld the fundamental assumptions, modes of thought, and scientific languages inherent to different disciplines. This collaborative effort can culminate in the development of computational models that simulate and elucidate the etiology and pathogenesis of diseases.

Words and Expressions

up-to-date　最新的

*You need to subscribe to those journals if you want to obtain **up-to-date** information about the public health study.*

genome　基因组

*The human **genome** consists of approximately 3 billion base pairs and contains the genetic information that shapes our biology.*

transcriptome　转录组

*The **transcriptome** analysis revealed significant changes in gene expression patterns associated with the disease, providing valuable insights into its molecular mechanisms.*

proteome　蛋白质组

*The study of the **proteome** allowed researchers to identify specific protein markers associated with the early stages of the disease, offering potential targets for therapeutic intervention.*

metabolome　代谢组

*The **metabolome** is exquisitely sensitive to what people eat, where they live, what is the* *time, what is the season, their general health and even their mood.*

landmark 里程碑

*The discovery of antibiotics was a **landmark** in the field of medicine, revolutionizing the treatment of bacterial infections and saving countless lives.*

primary 原发性的

*It is not the **primary** tumor that kills, but secondary growths elsewhere in the body.*

alteration 改动, 更改, 改变

*The change in the character of a cell is determined by the **alterations** in genetics and epigenomics.*

multidisciplinary （涉及）多门学科的, 有关各种学问的, 多专业的

*Data mining is a **multidisciplinary** field incorporating many techniques.*

petabyte 拍字节或千万亿字节或千 T 字节（较高级的储存单位）

*The new maximum pp size provides an architectural support for 256 **petabyte** disks.*

aneuploidy ［遗］非整倍性; 异倍体性; 异倍性

*One measure of malignancy is **aneuploidy** by flow cytometry.*

phosphoprotein 磷蛋白质

*The aim is to investigate if there are disease-specific mutations within the dentin **phosphoprotein** in two dentinogenesis imperfecta type Ⅱ families, and analyze the nucleotide polymorphism in the DPP region.*

taxonomy 分类学; 分类法

Taxonomy is the practice and science of categorization or classification. In biology, taxonomy is the scientific study of naming, defining and classifying groups of biological organisms based on shared characteristics.

histology 组织学

Histology is the study of the microanatomy of cells, tissues, and organs as seen through a microscope.

pathology 病理学; 病状; 精神异常; 社会异常; 语言异常

*The objective is to explore the clinical **pathology** of ovarian dysgerminoma.*

embryonic 胚胎的; 胚的; 初期的

Embryonic stem cells (ES cells or ESCs) are pluripotent stem cells derived from the inner cell mass of a blastocyst, an early-stage pre-implantation embryo.

progenitor 祖先; 原著; 起源

*Pluripotent stem cells are capable of self-renewal to generate themselves and are capable of dividing into both bioloid and lymphoid **progenitor** cells.*

abuse 滥用, 虐待

*The **abuse** of prescription opioids has become a significant concern in the field of medicine, leading to addiction and adverse public health consequences.*

oncogenic 致瘤的; 瘤原性的

*Seropositivity rates for non-oncogenic or **oncogenic** HPV types did not differ between cases and controls.*

metastases   转移（metastasis 的复数）

Metastases, the spread of cancer from one organ or part of the body to another, often pose significant challenges in the field of medicine, requiring advanced treatments and interventions.

stratify   分层

*In the field of medicine, researchers aim to **stratify** patients into distinct risk groups based on genetic factors to develop personalized treatment plans.*

stromal   基质的

***Stromal cells** are connective tissue cells of any organ, for example in the uterinemucosa (endometrium), prostate, bone marrow, and the ovary where a **stromal tumor** is a tumor that arises in the supporting connective tissue of an organ.*

mesenchymal   间叶细胞的；由间叶细胞组成的；间叶细胞样的

*These observations exhibited an obvious biphasic differentiated (epithelial and **mesenchymal**) nature of tumor cells, and indicated that adenomatoid tumors were of mesothelial origin.*

integrative   综合的；一体化的

*It indicates only correct **integrative** treatment can improve survival rates.*

dedifferentiation   特殊细胞形态的消失

*A **dedifferentiation** of mitochondria and plastids in structure in microspore mother cells was observed at from diplonema/diakinesis to metaphase I, then a redifferentiation at dyad stage.*

paradigm   范例；词形变化表

*The introduction of precision medicine marked a significant **paradigm** shift in the field of medicine, emphasizing individualized treatment based on a patient's genetic makeup.*

momentous   重大的，严重的

*The **momentous** news was that war had begun.*

simulate   模仿；假装；冒充

*The PMK programing controller is used to **simulate** the process control system and adjust the parameters of the controller in the extractive tower.*

standardization   标准化

*Nowadays, more and more people eat characteristic healthy food like hoecake with strengthened nutrition consciousness. To ensure the **standardization** of products, the standard of enterprise was drawn.*

unification   统一，联合，一致

*Tasting ideal is the **unification** of representationalism and abstraction of finiteness and infinity.*

fuse   熔化；融合；合并；保险丝，熔丝；导火线；引信

*You'll blow a **fuse** if you put the electric heater and the cooker on at the same time.*

experimental   实验性的，试验性的

*For the time being, however, immunotherapy is still in its **experimental** stages.*

theoretical   理论的；理论上存在的，假设的

*It's a **theoretical** matter as well as a practical one.*

cooperation 合作, 协作; 协助, 配合

*The technical **cooperation** and cultural exchanges between the two countries are daily on the increase.*

Language Point

Machine Learning 机器学习

Machine learning (ML) is a branch of artificial intelligence (AI) focused on the development of computer algorithms capable of self-improvement through experience and data utilization. ML algorithms create predictive or decision-making models based on training data, eliminating the need for explicit programming. These algorithms find applications in various fields, including medicine, email filtering, speech recognition, and computer vision, particularly in scenarios where the creation of conventional algorithms for complex tasks is impractical or unachievable.

*An illustrative case highlighting the capacity of **machine learning** to enhance disease diagnosis accuracy is found in medical image analysis, particularly in automating diabetic retinopathy screening.*

Multiomics 多组学

Multiomics, often referred to as multi-omics, integrative omics, "panomics," or 'pan-omics,' is a comprehensive biological analysis approach that involves the simultaneous study of multiple "omes" such as the genome, proteome, transcriptome, epigenome, metabolome, and microbiome. In essence, it leverages various omics technologies to collectively investigate life processes.

*In a **multiomics** study involving patients with uncharacterized Fanconi anaemia, DNA sequencing and array comparative genomic hybridization (aCGH) successfully identified the causal mutations, while RNA-seq offered evidence of pathogenicity for certain unexpected variants.*

EXERCISES

Task 1: Vocabulary Application

Fill in the blanks with the words given below. Change the form where necessary.

> **multidisciplinary; embryonic; progenitor; paradigm; metastasis; landmark; taxonomy; oncogenic; stratify; proteome**

1. The introduction of telemedicine as a primary mode of healthcare delivery during the COVID-19 pandemic challenged the traditional of _____ in-person medical consultations.

2. We know that Hepatitis C virus is an _____ virus. It's a cancer-causing virus and together with HIV may increase the risk of cancers.

3. In 2011, they released a _____ study titled "Academically Adrift," which documented the lack of intellectual growth experienced by many people enrolled in college.

4. Kevin Lou, the CEO of Mount Elizabeth hospital in Singapore, said that _____ team of specialists have been working tirelessly to treat the young woman.

5. These are stem cells and the more developed neural _____ cells.

6. _____ is the major cause of death from cancer.

7. The _____ is the library of information that creates proteins.

8. _____ stem cells have been the focus in tissue engineering, developmental biology, drug development and gene research.

9. _____ is a word describing to a process of placing things in groups based on their qualities.

10. We can use genetics to _____ patients in clinical development.

Task 2: Writing

For this part, you are given 30 minutes to compose an essay on the topic: Systems Epidemiology in Cancer. You should write at least 120 words, and base your composition on the outline below:

1) Compare the traditional approach to cancer epidemiology studies with a systems design.

2) Explain the advantages of employing systems epidemiology in cancer research?

Task 3: Oral Presentation

Systems epidemiology holds promise in elucidating the etiology of prevalent chronic non-communicable diseases, including cardiovascular conditions, diabetes, cancer, and more. Provide a concise summary of a study related to one of these diseases, outlining its current research status and highlighting forthcoming challenges.

Learning Garden

Mathematical Methods in Systems Epidemiology

Network analysis methods serve as the computational backbone for integrating data and selecting biomarkers in systems epidemiology. Analyzing multiple omics data concurrently is inherently intricate. Recent years have witnessed the increasing application of various network analysis techniques. These include networking reasoning, which employs a statistical regression framework; pathway network analysis, rooted in biological hypotheses; and comprehensive network analysis, blending data-driven and hypothesis-driven approaches. Continuous refinement and innovation of advanced computational network analysis methods is ongoing. Notably, tools like Cytoscape software and STRING databases offer versatile resources for visualizing and analyzing omics data within biological networks. Moreover, transmission dynamic modeling plays a vital role in understanding infectious disease transmission. Despite these advances, the management of complex multi-layer, multi-omics data will necessitate further optimization in the future.

（刘斯洋、杜向军）

Unit 9　Major Public Health Emergencies and Responses

READING A

PREVIEW

What is a public health emergency? It is hard to define, because it includes not only infectious diseases that cause public health events but also widespread injuries, such as those caused by drugs or vehicle crashes. The definition of public health emergency cannot be limited only to-diseases but should include big events that affect people's health. The first reading below will provide you with some knowledge about public health emergencies.

Questions for Discussion

Q1: What is a public health emergency? What are the criteria for a satisfactory public health emergency response?

Q2: What are the extraordinary legal actions for officials to take when a public health emergency happens?

Text A

What is a Public Health Emergency?

On March 27, 2014, Massachusetts Governor Deval Patrick declared the state's opioid-addiction **epidemic** a public health emergency. The declaration **empowered** the Massachusetts public health commissioner to use emergency powers to expand access to naloxone, an opioid **antagonist** that can reverse overdoses; develop a plan to accelerate the mandatory use of prescription monitoring by physicians and **pharmacists**; and prohibit the prescribing and dispensing of hydrocodone-only medication (Zohydro, Zogenix), which had been recently approved by the Food and Drug Administration (FDA), amid much controversy. The governor also allocated $20 million for addiction treatment services.

The public health problem-the advent of a potentially dangerous new drug following 140 deaths due to **heroin** overdoses in 4 months and a 90% increase in unintentional opiate overdoses between 2000 and 2012-warranted a robust response. Nevertheless, Patrick's unusual invocation of emergency public health powers, which are traditionally reserved for infectious disease outbreaks, natural disasters, or acts of terrorism, offers an opportunity to consider some important questions. Should **widespread** injuries caused by opiates or motor **vehicle** crashes be viewed as public health emergencies? Should chronic health conditions such as **hypertension** or **obesity** be similarly categorized? When should normal lawmaking processes, and the typical rights afforded to individuals and entities, be suspended to protect public health?

State laws providing public health emergency powers permit designated officials-typically governors and their top health officers-to take extraordinary legal actions. These laws provide flexibility in responding to emergency situations where adherence to ordinary legal standards and processes could cost lives.

State laws vary in their definitions of "emergency" or "disaster". Many refer to an occurrence or imminent threat of widespread or severe damage, injury, or loss of life or property resulting from a natural **phenomenon** or human act (see table 1). Some mention only the magnitude of the potential harm without specifying its source. Others, including the Massachusetts law, provide no definition, leaving it to the governor to determine what constitutes an emergency.

Once a public health emergency is declared, designated officials can harness powers that are typically unavailable without legislative approval, by issuing emergency orders. These expansive powers may include deploying military personnel, commandeering property, restricting freedom of movement, halting business operations, and suspending civil rights and **liberties**. Emergency orders can also tap resources reserved for the proverbial rainy day.

Emergency powers largely sit outside the ordinary structures of checks and balances. Even when time-limited, they are generally renewable at the governor's discretion; only some of them can be terminated by the legislature (see Table 1).

The spirit of emergency-powers laws seems to enshrine three key **criteria** for suspending normal lawmaking processes: the situation is **exigent**, the anticipated or potential harm would be calamitous, and the harm cannot be avoided through ordinary procedures. The archetypal scenario is the sudden outbreak of a highly communicable, lethal disease -such as the unlikely event of an Ebola outbreak in a U.S. city -when immediate action is required to avert catastrophe. In such circumstances, acute concern for public health is believed to outweigh substantial trade-offs of values we ordinarily hold dear, including individual autonomy, due process, and democratic lawmaking.

Table 1. Illustrative State Laws on Emergency Powers for Public Health

State	Statute	Definition of Emergency or Disaster	Key Executive Powers	When Powers End
Indiana	Emergency Management and Disaster Law	Occurrence of imminent threat of widespread or severe damage, injury, or loss of life or property resulting from any natural phenomenon or human act, including epidemic and public health emergency	Act as militia commander-in-chief; suspend laws relating to the normal conduct of state business; use all available government resources; commandeer or use private property; control freedom of movement relating to evacuation and the disaster area; suspend or limit the sale, dispensing, or transportation of alcohol, explosives, and combustibles; and appropriate emergency or contingency funds (General Assembly also plays a role in appropriations)	Earlier of termination by the governor or by concurrent resolution of General Assembly or passage of 30 days (unless renewed by governor)
Massachusetts	Declaration of Emergency Detrimental to the Public Health	Not defined	Public health commissioner can take action and incur liability necessary to maintain public health and prevent disease	On governor's declaration
Pennsylvania	Governor and Disaster Emergencies	Not defined	Act as military commander-in-chief; suspend laws relating to normal order of government business; use all available government resources; commandeer or use any private, public, or quasi-public property; control freedom of movement relating to evacuation and the disaster area; and suspend or limit the sale, dispensing or transportation of alcohol, firearms, explosives, and combustibles.	Earlier of termination by the governor or by concurrent resolution of General Assembly or passage of 90 days (unless renewed by governor)
Washington	Washington State Emergency Management Act	Events or set of circumstances that demand immediate action to preserve public health, protect life, protect property, or provide relief to any stricken community overtaken by such circumstances; or that reaches such a dimension or degree of destructiveness as to warrant the governor's declaring a state of emergency	Control freedom of movement of persons; exercise powers without regard to procedures and formalities of law; enter into contracts and incur obligations on behalf of the government; use existing government resources; and commandeer private services and equipment	When terminated by the governor after restoration of order in the affected area

Words and Expressions

epidemic 流行病；流行性的
A flu epidemic is sweeping through Moscow.

empower 授权，给（某人）……的权力
The courts were empowered to impose the death sentence for certain crimes.

antagonist 拮抗剂，对手
Effect of calcium antagonists on insulin resistance in aged patients with hypertension.

pharmacist 药剂师
We had to wait for the pharmacist to make up her prescription.

heroin 海洛因
Heroin is a powerful illegal drug made from morphine that some people take for pleasure and can become addicted to.

widespread 普遍的，广泛的
The plan received widespread support throughout the country.

vehicle 交通工具，车辆，用以表达想法、情感的载体、方式方法
A vehicle is a machine such as a car, bus, or truck which has an engine and is used to carry people from place to place.
You can use vehicle to refer to something that you use in order to achieve a particular purpose.

hypertension 高血压
He suffered from hypertension and accompanying heart problems.

obesity 肥胖，肥胖症
Current thinking holds that obesity is more a medical than a psychological problem.

flexible 灵活的，能适应新情况的，易变通的
We should stick to the principles and be flexible as well.

phenomenon 现象
Science may be able to provide some explanations of paranormal phenomena.

liberty 自由
The right to vote should be a liberty enjoyed by all.

criteria 标准，准则
No candidate fulfills all the criteria for this position.

exigent 急迫的，催促的，紧急的
It is exigent to research and develop novel optical probes.

Language Points

addiction treatment 戒毒治疗

Drug addiction is a chronic disease characterized by compulsive, uncontrollable drug seeking and use despite harmful consequences and changes in the brain, which can be long-lasting. These changes in the brain can lead to harmful behaviors seen in people who use drugs. Drug addiction is also a relapsing disease. Drug treatment is intended to help addicted individuals stop compulsive drug seeking and use. Treatment can occur in a variety of settings, take many different forms, and last for different lengths of time. Because drug addiction is typically a chronic disorder characterized by occasional relapses, a short-term, one-time treatment is usually not sufficient. For many people, treatment is a long-term process that involves multiple interventions and regular monitoring.

*Her family arranged a comprehensive **addiction treatment** plan for her, including counseling, medication therapy, and rehabilitation programs, to help her overcome her alcohol dependence and rebuild a healthy life.*

EXERCISES

Task 1: Vocabulary Application

Fill in the blanks with the words given below. Change the form where necessary.

epidemic; antagonist; pharmacist; heroin; hypertension; obese; flexible; liberty; harness; legislative

1. _____ are required by law to give the medicine prescribed by the doctor.
2. Improving _____ control by home blood pressure telemonitoring system.
3. Your _____ is your opponent or enemy.
4. If someone is _____, they are extremely fat.
5. He systematically abused his body with _____ and cocaine.
6. _____ is the freedom to live your life in the way that you want, without interference from other people or the authorities.
7. _____ means that a large number of cases of a particular disease happen at the same time in a particular community.
8. Something or someone that is _____ can change easily and adapt to different conditions and circumstances as they occur.
9. Once a public health emergency is declared, designated officials can _____ powers that are typically unavailable without _____ approval, by issuing emergency orders.

Task 2: Writing

Letters to the public health media are effective tools of public health advocacy because they allow access to a general audience. For this part, you are allowed to write a letter to express your views on the necessity of taking extraordinary legal actions when a public health emergency occurs. You should write at least 150 words but no more than 300 words.

Task 3: Oral Presentation

Describe a public health event you have experienced. Clearly express the beginning time and the place of this incident, the reason for it, the measures taken by the government at that time, and the result. Summarize the event, give your personal views, and put forward some constructive suggestions.

READING B

PREVIEW

There are public health emergencies of all kinds, each of which demands a specific response. Public health emergency preparedness, however, always requires the same basic steps: researching the problem, communicating prevention information and activities, and disseminating care and recovery information. What differences exist in China? What adjustments and changes has China made regarding public health emergencies and res-ponses?

Questions for Discussion

Q1: What achievements has China made in public health emergency response?

Q2: What plan did China make based on the current situation for the future?

Text B

Public Health Emergency Response in China

Public health emergencies refer to major epidemics of infectious diseases, unexplained mass psychogenic illness, major food poisoning, occupational poisoning, and other events that have a serious impact on public health. According to the *Emergency Response Low of the People's Republic of China,* public health **emergencies are categorized into** four levels for their respective responses: extremely serious (level Ⅰ), serious (level Ⅱ), relatively serious (level Ⅲ), and common (level Ⅳ), based on the characteristics, the **hazard** degree, and the scope of the event. Considering response capability, vulnerability, secondary **disaster**, social concern, and other factors, the one-to-one correspondence between severity level and response level does not work sometimes. Therefore, different regions have different responses to public health emergencies in China.

The basic work of the public health emergency system is to respond. And the core of that is the response capability. Since the eleventh five-year plan, China's public health emergency system has experienced three steps in ten years. The first step is the construction of "one case, three systems" (a plan, an organization system, a legal system, and a working system). The secondary step of system construction is maintenance and improvement. The third step is standardization. After these three steps, a new pattern of the public health system has been formed, which is reflected in four aspects. The organization of public health emergencies has grown from scratch. The management of it has changed from decentralized to centralized. The method of it has changed from relying on experience to being based on the law. The working mode of it has changed from heavy disposal to equal **emphasis** on prevention and disposal. And the working mechanism of it has changed from single-department response to multi-department coordination. The response to major public health emergencies includes prevention, preparation, **monitoring**, early warning, reporting, response, disposal, recovery, and reconstruction. It involves many disciplines such as medicine, epidemiology, **sociology**, management, and communication. It needs the leadership of the government, the assistance of departments, and the participation of the whole society.

The key to effective public health emergency response is to prioritize both prevention and disposal equally. The core of that is to protect public health and life safety to the greatest extent and maintain the **harmony** and stability of society. At present, our system and capacity-building are not **compatible** with social and economic development, the global public health and safety situation, as well as the needs for people's health and safety. We must make up for the shortcomings in the area of public health and improve our ability to deal with major public health events. Achieving the goal requires us to focus on the system construction, and then, enhance that. Then, we should reform and improve the disease prevention and control system, improve the public health service system, strengthen the construction of public health teams, and enhance the collaborative mechanism for the study, evaluation, decision-making, and prevention and control of major public health risks. Moreover, we need to reform the prevention, control, and treatment system for a major public health emergency, to improve the emergency response mechanism, enhance the prevention and control politics and emergency treatment mode, and establish the treatment mechanism for that at different degrees, levels, and diversions. We need to improve the medical **insurance** and relief system for major diseases, explore the establishment of an exemption system for medical expenses for special groups and specific diseases, coordinate the use of basic medical insurance funds and public health service funds, increase the proportion of payments to grass-roots medical institutions, and realize the effective connection between public health services and medical services. We should unify the emergency material support system, optimize the production capacity support and regional layout of important emergency materials, and improve the connection between procurement, supply, and use. We should build a systematic, scientific, standardized, and effective legal system for epidemic prevention and control, comprehensively strengthen, and improve the construction of relevant laws and regulations in public health and strengthen the guarantee of the rule of law in public health.

Words and Expressions

emergency　突发事件, 紧急情况
*The government has declared a state of **emergency** following the earthquake.*

hazard　危险; 危害; 冒失地提出; 冒……的风险; 使处于危险
*Growing levels of pollution represent a serious health **hazard** to the local population.*

disaster　灾难, 灾祸, 灾害, 不幸
*Losing your job doesn't have to be such a **disaster**.*

emphasis　强调, 重视, 重要性
*We provide all types of information, with an **emphasis** on legal advice.*

monitor　班长, 监视器; 监视, 检查
*If you **monitor** something, you regularly check its development or progress and sometimes comment on it.*

epidemiology　流行病学
***Epidemiology** is a branch of medical science dealing with the transmission and control of disease*

sociology　社会学
***Sociology** is the study of society or of the way society is organized.*

harmony　融洽, 和睦

*If people are living in **harmony** with each other, they are living together peacefully rather than fighting or arguing.*

compatible　可共用的, 兼容的, 可共存的

*In a large city, you're almost certain to find a physician with whom you are **compatible** and feel comfortable.*

insurance　保险

***Insurance** is an arrangement in which you pay money to a company, and they pay money to you if something unpleasant happens to you, for example, if your property is stolen or damaged, or if you get a serious illness.*

Language Points

public health emergency　公共卫生事件

A public health emergency is a defined as "an occurrence or imminent threat of an illness or health condition, caused by bio terrorism, epidemic or pandemic disease, or an infectious agent or biological toxin, that poses a substantial risk to humans by either causing a significant number of human fatalities or permanent or long-term disability."

*The government declared a **public health emergency** in response to the rapid spread of a contagious disease, implementing measures to protect the population and contain the outbreak.*

one-to-one correspondence　一一对应

Matching one item to one corresponding item (or number).

*There is no simple **one-to-one correspondence** between optical depth and surface horizontal visibility.*

multi-departments　多个部门、跨部门

Of or pertaining to multiple departments.

*The rapid development of Internet technology, computer science, and software technology provides the possibility of **multi-departments** management and efficiency improvement.*

EXERCISES

Task 1: Vocabulary Application

Fill in the blanks with the words given below. Change the form where necessary.

> emergency; monitor; epidemiology; disaster; compatible; discipline; contemporary; avenue; morbidity; longevity

1. _____ is a sudden event, such as an accident or a natural catastrophe, that causes great damage or loss of life.

2. Their brains are scanned so that researchers can _____ the progress of the disease.

3. _____ is the method used to find the causes of health outcomes and diseases in populations.

4. If two people are _____, they can have a good relationship because they have similar ideas, interests, etc.

5. An _____ is an unexpected and difficult or dangerous situation, especially an accident, which happens suddenly, and requires quick action to deal with it.

6. It involves many _____ such as medicine, epidemiology, sociology, management, and communication.

7. The complexity of many _____ health problems requires multiple _____ of attack.

8. Even though the clinical care system has begun to focus more on reducing _____ and retaining function well into old age, large disparities in _____ persist.

Task 2: Writing

In the simulation scenario, there is an outbreak in a big city. Now you need to write a press release to explain the epidemic to the public. What aspects are you going to describe? You should write at least 150 words but no more than 300 words.

Task 3: Oral Presentation

In the simulation scenario, another epidemic outbreaks in a big city. If you are asked to respond to public health emergencies, what aspects do you plan to prepare? Please clearly express your point of view and explain why.

Learning Garden

The Secretary of Health and Human Services (HHS)

The Secretary of Health and Human Services (HHS) leads all Federal public health and medical responses to public health and medical emergencies covered by the National Response Framework. A number of national strategies and presidential directives establish HHS as the leading federal department responsible for protecting the health of the civilian population against both intentional, accidental, or naturally occurring threats. Additionally, *HHS Strategic Plan 2010-2015* calls for reducing the occurrence of infectious diseases, protecting Americans' health and safety during emergencies, and fostering resilience in response to emergencies; these goals are also reflected in particular strategic initiatives set by the secretary. Effectively fulfilling this responsibility and achieving these goals requires the coordination of medical countermeasure-related activities occurring across multiple federal departments. To provide this coordination, HHS established the Public Health Emergency Medical Countermeasures Enterprise (PHEMCE) in July 2006 to coordinate federal efforts aimed at enhancing civilian preparedness from a medical countermeasure perspective.

（冯铁建、孔令杰）

Reference：

HAFFAJEE R , PARMET W E , MELLO M M .What is a public health "Emergency"?[J]. The New England journal of medicine, 2014(11):371.

Unit 10 Prevention and Control of Pathogens and Infectious Diseases

READING A

PREVIEW

Most pandemics such as severe acute respiratory syndrome (SARS), human immunodeficiency virus/acquired immune deficiency syndrome (HIV/AIDS), and avian influenza, are caused by viruses, and are driven to emerge by behavioral, ecological, or socioeconomic changes. Despite their substantial effects on global public health and growing understanding of the process by which they emerge, no pandemic has been predicted before infecting human beings. Therefore, prevention and control strategies after the emergence of pathogens are still the main means to deal with infectious diseases. We review what is known about the pathogens that emerge, the hosts that they originate in, and the factors that drive their emergence, and list a series of prevention and control strategies that could help to overcome these challenges.

Questions for Discussion

Q1: What is the significance of the prevention and control of infectious diseases?

Q2: What are the main strategies for the prevention and control of infectious diseases?

Text A

The History of Infectious Diseases and their Prevention and Control Measures

Newly **emerging** (and **re-emerging**) infectious diseases have been threatening humans since the neolithic revolution, 12,000 years ago, when human **hunter-gatherers** settled into villages to domesticate animals and cultivate crops. These early stages of domestication marked mankind's initial steps towards systematic and widespread manipulation of nature. Ancient emerging **zoonotic** diseases with deadly consequences include **smallpox**, **falciparum malaria**, **measles**, and bubonic/**pneumonic plague**. Some notable examples include the Justinian Plague (541 AD) and the Black Death (1348 AD), both of which claimed a significant number of lives in the "known" world, i.e., the world known to those whose recordings of virus survive, predominantly in Asia, the Middle East, and Europe.

Only a century ago, the 1918 influenza pandemic killed 50 million or more people, making it apparently the **deadliest** event in recorded human history. The HIV/AIDS pandemic, recognized in 1981, has so far killed at least 37 million. Moreover, the past decade has witnessed **unprecedented** outbreaks of pandemic: H1N1 "swine" influenza (2009), chikungunya (2014), and Zika (2015), as well as Ebola fever emerging like a pandemic across large parts of Africa (2014).

Since there are four endemic coronaviruses that circulate globally in humans, it can be inferred that coronaviruses emerged and spread pandemically prior to the recognition of viruses as human pathogens. In 2002-2003, the severe acute respiratory syndrome (SARS) coronavirus (SARS-CoV) emerged from an animal host, most likely a civet cat, causing a near-pandemic before being controlled through public health control measures. Middle East respiratory syndrome (MERS) coronavirus (MERS-CoV), related to SARS-CoV, emerged into humans from dromedary camels in 2012, but has since been transmitted inefficiently among humans. The causes of this new and dangerous situation are multifaceted, complex, and deserving of serious examination.

When thinking about these recent infectious disease emergences, it is necessary to first consider currently existing infectious diseases that emerged in the past and subsequently became endemic (prevalent in humans) or enzootic (prevalent in animals). Such existing diseases may provide important clues about the mechanisms of disease emergence and persistence and why thus far we have been largely unable to prevent and control many of them.

The fact that many past emerging infectious **microbes** and viruses (hereafter grouped together as "microbes") have adapted to stable **co-existence** with humans is evidenced by the presence of endogenous **retroviruses** in human DNA and by **latently** infecting **herpes viruses** such as herpes simplex (HSV), cytomegalovirus (CMV), Epstein-Barr virus (EBV), and varicella-zoster virus (VZV). VZV, for example, is a highly cytolytic, highly contagious, and potentially fatal virus that has adapted to **long-term survival** in human populations via a complex survival mechanism. Unlike other highly contagious human-adapted respiratory viruses, such as measles - whose survival requires very large populations in order to avoid exhausting **susceptible persons** - VZV establishes latent non-cytolytic infections in human ganglia, **periodically** reactivating into an infectious/cytolytic form (zoster) that can be transmitted-even in populations without circulating varicella ("chicken pox") - to new birth cohorts of susceptible persons to be manifested as highly contagious varicella.

Human infectious agents such as retroviruses, herpesviruses, and many others tell us that long-ago emergences of certain diseases can result in long-term microbial survival by co-opting certain of our genetic, cellular, and immune mechanisms to ensure their continuing transmission. In the **terminology** of British biologist Richard Dawkins, evolution occurs at the level of gene competition and we, phenotypic humans, are merely genetic "survival machines" in the competition between microbes and humans. It may be a matter of perspective who is in the evolutionary driver's seat. This perspective has implications for how we think about and react to emerging infectious disease threats.

From the human point of view, the fact that modern **endemic diseases** emerged and became established, at some unobserved time in the past (Table 1), and that some of these diseases survived by adopting complicated long-term survival strategies, provides a **compelling** rationale for dual strategies for immediate and long-term control. Firstly, in the immediate sense, it is important to **mitigate** the spread of infection, illness, and death. Secondly, it is critical to prevent the persistence of microbes that may lead to additional emergences that are **cumulatively** as deadly, or more so, than the original emergences. That viral genetic descendants of the 1918 influenza pandemic virus are still causing seasonal outbreaks throughout the world, and still killing cumulatively millions of people a century later, is a powerful reminder that single disease emergencies can have consequences beyond immediate **morbidity** and **mortality**. In the ancient ongoing struggle between microbes and man, genetically more **adaptable** microbes have the upper hand in consistently surprising us and often **catching us unprepared**.

The latest example of this is the SARS pandemic that emerged in 2003. However, these are undoubtedly significant undercounts, reflecting early and still problematic access to diagnostic testing coupled with incomplete diagnoses of fatal cases. Since SARS was caused by a novel virus that produced a spectrum of diseases with clinical, pathologic, and epidemiologic patterns never observed before, we gained insights only incrementally. In the future, we will be better able to compare and contrast SARS with other important emerging diseases. However, at present, we are still just entering a steep learning curve that will surely continue to surprise us as we struggle to control what is already among the deadliest pandemics of the past century.

Table 1. Emerging Infectious Diseases in History

Year	Name	Deaths	Comments
430 BCE	"Plague of Athens"	roughly 100,000	First identified trans-regional pandemic
541	Justinian plague (*Yersinia pestis*)	30-50 million	Pandemic; killed half of world population
1340s	"Black Death" (*Yersinia pestis*)	roughly 50 million	Pandemic; killed at least a quarter of world population
1494	Syphilis (*Treponema pallidum*)	>50,000	Pandemic brought to Europe from the Americas
c. 1500	Tuberculosis	High millions	Ancient disease; became pandemic in Middle Ages
1520	*Hueyzahuatl* (*Variola major*)	3.5 million	Pandemic brought to New World by Europeans
1793-1798	"The American plague"	roughly 25,000	Yellow fever terrorized colonial America
1832	2nd cholera pandemic (Paris)	18,402	Spread from India to Europe/Western Hemisphere
1918	"Spanish" influenza	roughly 50 million	Led to additional pandemics in 1957, 1968, 2009
1976-2020	Ebola	15,258	First recognized in 1976; 29 regional epidemics to 2020
1981	Acute hemorrhagic conjunctivitis	rare deaths	First recognized in 1969; pandemic in 1981
1981	HIV/AIDS	roughly 37 million	First recognized 1981; ongoing pandemic
2002	SARS	813	Near-pandemic
2009	H1N1 "swine flu"	284,000	5th influenza pandemic of century
2014	Chikungunya	uncommon	Pandemic, mosquito-borne
2015	Zika	roughly 1,000?[*]	Pandemic, mosquito-borne

[*]Zika mortality has not been fully established. Most deaths are fetal or related to outcomes of severe congenital infections.

With the development and progress of medicine, **vaccines** and **antibiotics** have emerged as powerful tools for humans to fight pathogens and infectious diseases.

Since Edward Jenner developed the first vaccine to prevent smallpox infections to this day, in the course of more than two hundred years, the development of vaccines has undergone many **revolutions**, and corresponding research results have been applied to resist diseases and protect human health. Today, the application of vaccines has enabled some serious infectious diseases to be effectively controlled or eliminated.

The discovery of antibiotics is of **epoch-making** significance and completely reversed the passive situation in which human beings were helpless and waiting to die in the face of bacterial diseases. During the First World War, the number of soldiers who died from wound infections was much higher than the number of soldiers killed on the **battlefield**. At that time, people's lives were extremely **fragile**. **Tetanus**, **sepsis**, **streptococcal** infection, and even minor skin **abrasions** may cause damage. After 20 years, during the Second World War, the discovery and application of antibiotics saved the lives of **countless** soldiers. After the war, we **ushered** in a golden age of antibiotics. However, everything stems from penicillin-one of the greatest discoveries of the 20th century-making antibiotic drugs a powerful tool for people to fight infectious diseases.

In the current prevention and control of infectious diseases, vaccines activate the body's immunity and play a role in preventing pathogen infections; and anti-infective drugs can effectively inhibit or kill pathogens in the host, contributing to the control of epidemics caused by infectious diseases. Therefore, vaccines and anti-infective drugs, as important tools for humans to against emerging (and re-emerging) infectious diseases, will play an increasingly important role in the prevention and control of infectious diseases in the future.

Words and Expressions

emerge 浮现；变得显眼（或突出）；（事实、情况）被知晓

*Asia's **emerging** economies will be on a self-sustaining cycle of growth.*

re-emerge 再次浮现，东山再起

*We will witness its **re-emergence** in a different manner in the upcoming days.*

hunter-gatherers 采集狩猎的人

*Attempts to identify New Guinean's **hunter-gatherers** face the well-known difficulty of defining what constitutes a hunter-gather group.*

smallpox ［内科］天花

*If **smallpox** occurred in your community, about 30 percent of the people that acquire the disease would die from it.*

falciparum malaria ［内科］恶性疟；热带疟

*WHO's treatment policy is to treat all cases of uncomplicated **falciparum malaria** with* *artemisinin combination therapy (ACTs).*

measles ［内科］麻疹；风疹

*About 93 percent of U.S. residents are immune to **measles** either because they were vaccinated or they had the disease as a child.*

pneumonic plague ［内科］肺炎性鼠疫

*According to WHO, **pneumonic plague** is one of the deadliest infectious diseases, capable of killing humans within 24 hours of infection.*

deadliest 最致命的

*Meanwhile, the **deadliest** strains of the virus perished with their hosts as natural selection favored strains that could infect hosts but not kill them.*

unprecedented 前所未有的，史无前例的

*The mission has been hailed as an **unprecedented** success.*

microbe 细菌，［微］微生物

*These **microbes** enable the soil to have more nitrogen, which is essential for plant growth, and they remain quite active during the winter.*

co-existence 共生；共存性

***Co-existence** is not only a biological phenomenon, but also a social phenomenon.*

retrovirus ［病毒］逆转录酶病毒

*HIV is a special type of virus known as a **retrovirus**.*

long-term survival 长期存活

*In vitro, virus in the coagulation of blood can not be **long-term survival**.*

susceptible persons 易感人群

*The cold air is blowing from the north, for influenza **susceptible persons**, the strengthening of routine influenza prevention measures is particularly important.*

latent 潜在的

*These children have a huge reserve of **latent** talent.*

periodically 定期地；周期性地；偶尔；间歇

*For reasons not fully understood, the field itself reverses **periodically** every million years or so.*

herpesvirus ［病毒］疱疹病毒

*Mice infected with a **herpesvirus** generally develop keratitis, a degenerative disease affecting part of the eye.*

terminology 术语，术语学

*Standard medical **terminology** uses jaundice for a symptom yellow discolouration of skin.*

endemic diseases ［内科］地方病

*At the same time, China's major infectious diseases, **endemic diseases** prevention and control efforts have also been strengthened.*

compelling 令人信服的，有说服力的

*In this case, the argument for strict regulation is **compelling**.*

mitigate 缓和,减轻

*We will have to **mitigate** and adapt to avert the most extreme scenario.*

cumulatively 累积地;渐增地

***Cumulatively** 822 cases, including 29 deaths, were reported in Mexico.*

adaptable 适合的;能适应的;可改变的

*Human beings are infinitely **adaptable**.*

catch us unprepared 让我们措手不及

*In 2020, the virus descended swiftly onto the world, **catching us** unaware and **unprepared**.*

vaccine 疫苗

*Twelve potential **vaccines** are currently being tested on human volunteers.*

antibiotics [药]抗生素

***Antibiotics** should be used to clear up the infection.*

ancestor [生物]祖先,上代

*Our **ancestors** merely made use of their hands to change nature.*

revolution 彻底变革,革命

*A resident of his neighborhood had let off fireworks to celebrate the **revolution**.*

epoch-making 划时代的;开新纪元的

*The use of the Internet is an **epoch-making** event.*

battlefield 战场;沙场

*The castle stands on the site of an ancient **battlefield**.*

fragile 易碎的,易损的

*Because of the extreme cold, the Antarctic is a uniquely **fragile** environment.*

Tetanus [内科]破伤风;强直

***Tetanus** is an acute bacterial disease caused by clostridium tetani.*

sepsis 败血症,[医]脓毒病;腐败作用

*The catalog of protein molecules associated with **sepsis** is extensive.*

streptococcal 链球菌所导致的;链状球菌的

*The relative study between psoriasis and **streptococcal** infection is one of the hot spots these years.*

abrasion [皮肤]擦伤;[机][口腔]磨损

*The bacteria get into humans through **abrasions** in the skin.*

countless 无数的,数不尽的

*The new treatment could save Emma's life and the lives of **countless** others.*

usher 引导,招待;迎接;开辟;引座员

*She **ushered** her guests to their seats.*

Language Point

newly emerging (and re-emerging) infectious diseases 新发(再发)传染病

There are many factors involved in the emergence of new infectious diseases or the re-emergence of "old" infectious diseases. Some result from natural processes, such as the evolution of pathogens over time, while many others are a result of human behavior and practices.

Newly emerging and re-emerging infectious diseases *are both the epidemiologists need to pay close attention to.*

EXERCISES

Task 1: Vocabulary Application

Fill in the blanks with the words given below. Change the form where necessary.

zoonotic; streptococcal; mortality; fragile; mitigate; re-emerging; periodically; susceptible persons; cumulatively; microbes

1. At first, the drug does no harm, but _____ its effects are bad.

2. Markets crowded with domestic animals or wildlife are the perfect breeding ground for the spread of _____ diseases.

3. New challenges have arisen in the public health control of emerging and _____ infectious diseases.

4. For reasons not fully understood, the field itself reverses _____ every million years or so.

5. Recent studies suggested that erythromycin may be effective in prophylaxis against pertussis in exposed, _____.

6. Indirectly through inanimate fomites (objects). Examples are _____ infection, streptococcal infection, colds, hospital-acquired wound infections through use of improperly sterilized items.

7. Infant and maternal _____ rates went down 132 percent and 147 percent respectively.

8. The _____ economies of several southern African nations could be irreparably damaged.

9. The leases come with painstaking stipulations to _____ any possible environmental harm to species like the polar bear.

10. These _____ enable the soil to have more nitrogen, which plants need to live and they remain quite active during the winter.

Task 2: Writing

For this part, you are allowed 30 minutes to write a composition on the topic: newly emerging (and re-emerging) infectious diseases. You should write at least 120 words, and base your composition on the outline below:

1) The characteristics of infectious diseases.

2) The difference between newly emerging infectious diseases and re-emerging infectious diseases?

3) What are the main strategies to fight infectious diseases?

Task 3: Oral Presentation

Introduce an infectious disease and describe its prevention and control measures

READING B

PREVIEW

*Influenza is an infectious **respiratory** disease that, in humans, is caused by influenza A and influenza B viruses. It is typically characterized by annual **seasonal** epidemics, with sporadic pandemic outbreaks **involving** zoonotic strains of the influenza A virus. The World Health Organization (WHO) estimates that annual epidemics of influenza result in approximately 1 billion infections, 3–5 million cases of severe illness and 300,000–500,000 deaths. The severity of a pandemic influenza depends on multiple factors, including the **virulence** of the pandemic virus strain and the level of **pre-existing** immunity. The most severe influenza pandemic occurred in 1918 and resulted in over 40 million deaths worldwide. Influenza vaccines are formulated every year to match the **circulating strains**, as they evolve **antigenically** owing to antigenic **drift**. Nevertheless, vaccine efficacy is not optimal and is **dramatically** low in the case of an antigenic mismatch between the vaccine and the circulating virus strain. **Antiviral** agents that target the influenza virus enzyme neuraminidase have been developed for prophylaxis and therapy. However, the use of these antivirals is still limited. Emerging approaches to combat influenza include the development of universal influenza virus vaccines that provide protection against antigenically distant influenza viruses, but these vaccines need to be tested in clinical trials to ascertain their effectiveness.*

Questions for Discussion

Q1: What are the epidemic characteristics of influenza?

Q2: Facing the flu epidemic, what preventive and control measures should be taken?

Text B

Prevention and Control of Influenza: Vaccines and Antiviral Drugs

Influenza is an infectious **respiratory** disease; in humans, it is caused by influenza A (genus influenzavirus A) and influenza B (genus influenzavirus B) viruses (influenzavirus C and influenzavirus D genera are also known). **Symptoms** associated with influenza virus infection vary from a mild respiratory disease confined to the upper respiratory tract, characterized by **fever**, **sore throat**, runny nose, **cough**, headache, muscle pain and fatigue to severe and in some cases lethal pneumonia owing to influenza virus or to secondary bacterial infection of the lower respiratory tract. Influenza virus infection can also lead to a wide range of non-respiratory complications in some cases-affecting the heart, central nervous system and other organ systems. Although characterized by annual **seasonal** epidemics, sporadic and **unpredictable** global pandemic outbreaks also occur that involve influenza A virus strains of zoonotic origin. Pandemic influenza occurs every 10–50 years and is characterized by the introduction of a new influenza A virus strain that is **antigenically** very different from previously circulating strains; the lack of pre-existing immunity in humans is often associated with the severity of the infection and an increase in mortality.

The major burden of disease in humans is caused by seasonal epidemics of influenza A and influenza B viruses, with most of the infections occurring in children, although most of the severe cases involve very young or elderly individuals. Currently, seasonal influenza A H1N1 and H3N2 circulate in humans, but from 1957 to 1968 the only human circulating influenza A viruses were influenza A H2N2 viruses. Before 1918, conclusive evidence of the circulating **subtypes** is not available. In addition to seasonal epidemics, the introduction of influenza A viruses from either **avian** or **swine** populations has led to four pandemics since 1918, with those viruses subsequently becoming seasonal epidemic strains in subsequent years. During pandemics, influenza viruses spread very quickly from the point of origin to the rest of the world in several waves during the year owing to the lack of pre-existing immunity, which could also contribute to increased virulence.

In 2009, the first influenza virus pandemic of this century was caused by a reassortant of a novel H1N1 influenza A virus that was previously circulating in pigs. Vaccines were not available on time to contain the first wave of infection. Current influenza antiviral adamantane drugs that target the viral M2 **ion channel** and inhibitors of NA enzymes have limitations, as viral **resistance** against M2 inhibitors is **prevalent** in the currently circulating human influenza A H1N1 and H3N2 strains; viruses resistant to the NA inhibitor oseltamivir have been prevalent among influenza A H1N1 strains since just before the 2009 pandemic. Intriguingly, the adamantane-resistant, oseltamivir-sensitive 2009 pandemic influenza A H1N1 viruses replaced the previously circulating oseltamivir-resistant, adamantane-sensitive seasonal influenza A H1N1 virus that circulated **globally** in 2008–2009. Although detection of the currently circulating influenza A H1N1 viruses harboring the *NA-H275Y* **mutation**, which imparts oseltamivir resistance, has been noted, emergence of resistance to NA inhibitors is not a major public health problem today. Current seasonal influenza vaccines have only suboptimal effectiveness across all age groups, particularly in elderly individuals (a high-risk group for severe influenza virus infection). Thus, there is a major need to better understand the biology of influenza virus infections to develop new and more-effective antiviral drugs and vaccines.

After the **causative** agent of influenza was identified to be a virus in the 1930s, attempts were made during World War Ⅱ to develop **inactivated** virus as a vaccine, which **culminated** in the licensing of the first influenza virus vaccine for the civilian population in 1945 in the United States. Unfortunately, it soon became clear that the vaccine did not protect well against new influenza virus strains. Specifically, the 1947 seasonal epidemic strain had changed sufficiently that the vaccines made with earlier circulating strains had lost their effectiveness. Although antigenic **shift** and antigenic drift in influenza viruses are recognized problems, the procedure to **manufacture** influenza virus vaccines has remained largely unchanged for many decades. The manufacture of influenza virus vaccines involves growing the virus in embryonated chicken eggs and inactivation using formalin (or another alkylating reagent).

In 2003, MedImmune (Gaithersburg, Maryland, USA) introduced the first live **attenuated** influenza virus vaccine (LAIV) licensed in the United States. This vaccine is based on the backbones of the influenza A/Ann Arbor/6/1960 and influenza B/Ann Arbor/1/1966 strains, through the passaging of the viruses at low temperature (25 °C). Cold-adapted influenza virus vaccines based on the same principle and developed by the Institute of Experimental Medicine have been successfully used in Russia since 1987. Seasonal vaccines are made by **reassortment** of the six internal RNA segments of the cold-adapted strain with the HA and NA RNA segments of the influenza virus strains specified by the health authorities for inclusion in the seasonal vaccines. Vaccine strain selection for both inactivated vaccines and LAIVs is based on the determination of the prevalence of recent human circulating strains by multiple laboratories engaged in a WHO-sponsored influenza surveillance program. LAIVs seem to have advantages in inducing **mucosal** and more broadly protective immune responses in infants and children than inactivated influenza virus preparations. However, studies with LAIVs in the United States have shown poor efficacy against the influenza A H1N1 component.

Another breakthrough for influenza vaccines came in 2013, when the FDA licensed Flublok (Protein Sciences Corporation, Meriden, Connecticut, USA), which is a product made exclusively using **recombinant** DNA technologies. For the quadrivalent product, four different baculoviruses expressing the HA of two types of influenza A viruses and the HA of two types of influenza B viruses are used to infect continuous insect cell lines; the HA proteins are then extracted and purified from the infected cells-a process that completely avoids the use of influenza viruses and embryonated eggs. Thus, there is now a faster start-up possible for vaccine manufacturing in cases of vaccine shortages or the emergence of novel pandemic strains. Furthermore, there is no need for time-consuming adaptations of the vaccine strains to increase yields in embryonated eggs or in tissue culture, as the recombinant baculoviruses express different HAs at comparable levels in insect cells.

The addition of adjuvants to inactivated influenza vaccines can improve vaccine efficacy, broaden and prolong protection, and provide dose-sparing benefits during years with vaccine shortages. In 2013, the FDA approved an **adjuvant** influenza vaccine for the prevention of pandemic influenza A H5N1. To increase the poor immunogenicity of inactivated influenza vaccines in elderly individuals, an unadjuvanted high-dose vaccine has also been developed and proven to decrease severe influenza virus infection outcomes compared with standard-dose vaccines. In addition, some available influenza vaccines are now tetravalent, incorporating both lineages of the influenza B virus. Thus, the variety of approved influenza virus vaccines has been dramatically increased in recent decades globally. However, all these available seasonal influenza virus vaccines still require annual **reformulation** to match antigenically circulating strains. In addition, the short duration of immunity is another major shortcoming of current vaccines.

Assays to **monitor** antigenicity of prior viruses are performed on a regular basis, generally by government laboratories. The antigenicity of a virus is detected by infecting naive ferrets with the cultured virus and collecting the sera 2-3 weeks later; the ability of the sera to inhibit hemagglutination compared against the current vaccine is monitored. Sera from an antigenically novel virus will show reduced hemagglutination inhibitory activity compared with previous virus strains, indicating antigenic drift and a potential vaccine mismatch.

In the absence of a universal vaccine that covers all possible strains and subtypes of influenza virus, many countries have implemented stockpiling vaccine programs to store vaccines against influenza virus strains with pandemic potential for emergency first responders in order to **alleviate** the problem imposed by the rapid spread of pandemic influenza. Despite the availability of seasonal and pandemic influenza vaccines, debate is ongoing as to the efficacy and effectiveness of these vaccines. Although different **methodologies**, variability in virulence among seasonal strains, fit or matching between the vaccine and circulating strains, as well as age differences among cohorts can make interpretation of results between studies difficult, most studies find a positive effect of vaccination on the overall health of vaccinated individuals. Nevertheless, many challenges still remain, including documented lack of efficacy of LAIVs in the United States in the past years, possible reduced vaccine efficacy with repeated annual immunizations, and problems associated with vaccine mismatches.

Together with vaccines, antiviral drugs play a vital part in the prevention and treatment of influenza virus infection and disease. In a normal influenza season, antiviral drugs are primarily used for treating patients who are severely ill, particularly those who have a **compromised** immune system. In a pandemic setting, especially in the period before a vaccine becomes available, antiviral drugs are essential for both treating patients who have been infected and preventing infection in individuals who have been exposed. Currently, there are two classes of approved drugs for influenza: the adamantanes and the NA inhibitors.

Amantadine and rimantadine are both orally administered drugs that target the M2 ion channel of influenza A viruses. However, these drugs are no longer globally recommended for clinical use because of widespread resistance among circulating influenza A viruses. By contrast, NA inhibitors target the enzymatic activity of the viral NA protein. Oseltamivir is delivered orally as the prodrug oseltamivir phosphate, which is converted to its active carboxylate form in the liver; zanamivir is inhaled as a **powder**; and peramivir is administered **intravenously**, which is important for **hospitalized patients**. All three drugs have received approval in the United States, Europe, Canada, Australia, Japan and Korea and act by mimicking the binding of **sialic acid** in the active site of NA on influenza A and influenza B viruses.

The emergence of **drug-resistant** viruses is a major challenge for the field of antiviral research. Adamantane resistance (conferred by an S31N mutation in the M2 protein) first emerged in influenza A H3N2 viruses in 2003 and became prevalent worldwide by 2008. The pandemic 2009 influenza A H1N1 virus, which is presently circulating as a seasonal H1N1 virus, is also resistant to the adamantanes, as its RNA segment of M gene was **inherited** from a virus that carried the S31N mutation.

Thus, since 2009, only the NA inhibitors have been able to provide protection, with the currently circulating human influenza A and influenza B viruses being generally sensitive to oseltamivir and zanamivir. However, the emergence of oseltamivir resistance is of particular concern for influenza A H1N1 viruses because it has happened in the past; in 2007, resistant influenza A H1N1 viruses began to circulate and quickly became dominant by the 2008-2009 season. The resistant **phenotype** is associated with an H275Y mutation in NA, and studies have shown that, in the background of other permissive mutations, H275Y-mutant viruses do not display any fitness **deficits**, which explains their ability to circulate so readily. Of note, these viruses remain sensitive to zanamivir. Perhaps fortuitously, the oseltamivir-resistant seasonal influenza A H1N1 virus was displaced by the introduction of the oseltamivir-sensitive pandemic influenza A H1N1 virus in 2009.

Since then, surveillance efforts have monitored NA inhibitor sensitivity closely and, although oseltamivir-resistant isolates of the 2009 influenza A H1N1 virus have been detected, these are primarily from patients undergoing therapy. **Susceptibility** to NA inhibitor is assessed by measuring NA enzyme inhibition in a functional assay using cultured virus. Alternatively, RT-PCR capable of detecting single nucleotide polymorphisms (or RT-PCR followed by sequencing) is used to detect known resistance mutations in NA, but the functional assay may be required if novel mutations are present.

There is a higher prevalence of resistant virus in children and individuals who are **immunocompromised**, which is believed to be related to higher **viral loads** and prolonged virus shedding in these individuals. Also, patients who have been hospitalized are more likely to receive longer treatment periods, which will increase the survival pressure on the virus and the likelihood that a resistant strain will emerge. Although this outcome may be predictable, oseltamivir resistance arose in 2007 seemingly in the absence of drug pressure; given the correct background of secondary mutations, the same outcome is a possibility for the current influenza A H1N1 virus. Oseltamivir resistance among influenza A H3N2 viruses and influenza B viruses has also been reported.

The **elimination** of adamantanes as clinical therapy, combined with concerns over increasing oseltamivir resistance illustrates the need for new influenza antiviral drugs. Several candidates are now in clinical trial, including additional NA inhibitors that can be delivered intravenously, such as **intravenous** formulations of zanamivir. Another NA inhibitor, laninamivir, has been approved for use in Japan; this drug is inhaled and long-acting and requires less frequent administration than oseltamivir or zanamivir.

Ideally, future influenza therapies will involve a cocktail of drugs with different mechanisms that should increase the barrier to resistance. Thus, drugs other than NA inhibitors are being clinically tested; within this pipeline are favipiravir (which is a polymerase inhibitor for several RNA viruses), pimodivir (which prevents the cap binding required for viral RNA transcription), baloxavir marboxil (an inhibitor of the cap-dependent endonuclease activity of the influenza viral polymerase) and nitazoxanide (an inhibitor of HA maturation). Baloxavir marboxil received approval in Japan in 2018. Favipiravir has also been approved in Japan since 2014, but only for release from government stockpile in the event of a novel strain being unresponsive to current agents. Treatment of patients who have been hospitalized with immune plasma or with hyperimmune immunoglobulin (pooled from plasma of donors with high titres of anti-influenza IgG) is also being clinically evaluated. In addition, several monoclonal antibodies against the conserved region of the HA stalk are also under clinical development for the treatment of severe influenza infection. Many more candidates are in preclinical development and will hopefully lead to improved options for influenza therapy in the future.

Words and Expressions

symptom ［医］症状
*One prominent **symptom** of the disease is progressive loss of memory.*

fever 发热；使发热，使激动不已
*His already infirm body was racked by a high **fever**.*

sore throat 咽喉痛
*The president declined to deliver the speech himself, on account of a **sore throat**.*

cough 咳嗽；发出咳嗽般的声音；咳嗽
*Contact your doctor if the **cough** persists.*

seasonal 季节性的，随季节变化的
*A monsoon is a **seasonal** wind that can bring in a large amount of rainfall.*

unpredictable 不可预知的
*A general trend can be recognized, but the details are usually **unpredictable**.*

antigenically 抗原性地
*In the present study, H9N2 viruses isolated from chicken, duck and other minor poultry were genetically and **antigenically** characterized.*

circulating 循环的；流通的

*The finding points to longstanding evidence that fiber may reduce **circulating** female hormone levels, which could explain the reduced risk.*

subtype 子类型，亚类

*Initial tests have identified the H5 **subtype** of avian influenza virus.*

avian 鸟的；鸟类的

*Wild birds have caught the canary pox virus, and penguins have been stricken by **avian** malaria.*

swine 猪

*I have family and friends who have had **swine** flu, though I doubt if they appear in the figures.*

strain 品种，类型

*Meanwhile, PG9 and PG16 can also be effective against multiple HIV viral **strains**, including those from the spread of AIDS in Africa, the most severe **strain**.*

pre-existing 现存的；已存的

*Her death is now thought to have been caused by this **pre-existing** disease.*

reassortment 重配

*The virus is produced by a **reassortment**, in which human-adapted H1N1 swaps genes with an H2N2 bird flu.*

prevalent 盛行的，普遍的

*Despite the fact that the disease is so **prevalent**, treatment is still far from satisfactory.*

mutation 突变；变化

*If a copy of a gene is a bit different from the original, that's called a genetic **mutation**.*

culminated （以……）结束，告终；到达顶点

*The sense of wrongs, the injustices, the oppression, extortion, and pillage of twenty years suddenly **culminated** and found voice in a raucous howl of execration.*

shift 改变，转变；（使）移动，（使）转移

*Avian influenza virus are highly labile, because of antigenic drift and antigenic **shift**.*

drift 流动，趋势；漂移，漂流

*It was apparent that the glaciation occurred in the relatively recent past because the **drift** was soft, like freshly deposited sediment.*

manufacture 大量制造；（用机器大量）生产，制造

*There are many procedures involved in the **manufacture** of food that result in greenhouse gases and other pollutants.*

involve 牵涉，涉及

*The treatment does not **involve** the use of any artificial drugs.*

attenuated （力量或效果）衰减的；使减弱；使变细

*They chose a bovine rotavirus because it grew well in culture and was thought to be naturally **attenuated** in humans.*

inactivated　灭活的

The **inactivated** protoplast fusion method was carried out to select new Bacillus thuringiensis strains.

mucosal　黏膜的

The **mucosal** adjuvants and delivery route were reviewed in this paper.

recombinant　（基因）重组的

The **recombinant** Bacmid containing fused ORF220 and EGFP gene was confirmed by PCR.

adjuvant　辅助的；佐药；辅助物

The purified recombinant major outer-membrane protein (MOMP) of Chlamydia psittaci (Cps) expressed in E. coli was mixed with oil **adjuvant**.

dramatically　剧烈地，明显地

The climate did not change **dramatically** from season to season.

reformulation　再形成

This paper reviews advances in researches of life cycle management using pharmaceutical **reformulation**.

alleviate　减轻，缓和

Several additional compounds were shown to **alleviate** proteotoxicity in worm models.

methodology　方法论，一套方法

This paper uses a new **methodology** for detecting this problem in this and related problems, exhibiting the property of "submodularity"

compromised　妥协的，妥协让步的；缺乏抵抗力的

It's possible that we all have **compromised** conversational intelligence.

ion channel　［物化］离子通道

Phospholamban pentamer can function as an **ion channel** and the mechanism is also unclear.

globally　全球地；全局地

Today, as the urban population explodes **globally**, cities are becoming more crowded.

powder　粉，粉末

It comes as a shock to us that some milk powder producers produce substandard milk **powder** which would bring harm to babies.

hospitalized　住院；入院就医

Most people do not have to be **hospitalized** for asthma or pneumonia.

sialic acid　唾液酸

Recently, **sialic acid** and derivates also play an important roles in cureing flu, neurogenic disease, inflammation and tumors.

drug-resistant　耐药的；抗药性的

HIV has been proven to possess the ability to mutate into **drug-resistant** forms.

inherited　遗传的；继承权的；继承（inherit 的过去分词）

*Doctors say the disease is probably **inherited** but not detectable at birth.*

phenotype ［遗］表型，表现型；显型

*The genetic mental retardation is the human **phenotype** blemish caused by injured DNA.*

deficit 亏损，赤字，不足额；缺乏，缺陷

*Therefore, the exploitation, research and utilization of chlorophyll-**deficit** mutant gene of rice have been highlighted.*

immunocompromised 免疫功能不全的

*CMV is usually seen in **immunocompromised** hosts and can be widespread in many organs.*

viral load 病毒载量

*The patients were found to have very low **viral loads** and stable CD4-cell counts after several years without therapy.*

elimination 消除，排除；淘汰；消灭

*We suspect that spending would come down through **elimination** of a lot of unnecessary or even dangerous tests and treatments.*

Language Point

viral load 病毒载量

Viral load tests measure the quantity of genetic material, commonly RNA, of a virus present in the blood. Several tests are typically conducted over an extended period, with initial measurements serving as the baseline and subsequent measurements being compared to these. Viral load measurements can differ daily, and therefore long-term trends are used to evaluate disease progression.

*The drugs can be used to reduce a woman's **viral load** effectively below detection.*

antigenic drift 抗原漂移

Antigenic drift refers to the gradual accumulation of point mutations during the annual circulation of influenza as a consequence of the high error rates associated with RNA-dependent RNA polymerase during virus replication.

*Avian influenza virus are highly labile, because of **antigenic drift** and antigenic shift.*

antigenic shift 抗原转变

Antigenic shift is a genetic alteration that occurs in an infectious agent, causing a dramatic change in an antigen protein, which stimulates the production of antibodies by the immune systems of humans and other animals.

*Pandemic influenza emerges as a result of major genetic changes, known as **antigenic shift**, occurring in influenza viruses.*

EXERCISES

Task 1: Vocabulary Application

Fill in the blanks with the words given below. Change the form where necessary.

alleviate; phenotype; inherit; resistance; adjuvant; reformulation; mutation; reassortment; symptom; antigenically

1. The genetic background of the disease _____ of the relationship is not over.

2. One prominent _____ of the disease is progressive loss of memory.

3. Scientists have genetically modified cotton to increase its _____ against insect pests.

4. We need to be aware of the risks and keep working to _____ the dangers.

5. _____ offers advantages over an original product in the improvement of efficacy and safety of drugs.

6. In the present study, H9N2 viruses isolated from chicken, duck and other minor poultry were genetically and _____ characterized.

7. Doctors say the disease is probably _____ but not detectable at birth.

8. The virus is produced by a _____, in which human-adapted H1N1 swaps genes with an H2N2 bird flu.

9. Once a lung cancer has been appropriately staged, primary and _____ therapeutic planning can commence.

10. Scientists have found a genetic _____ that appears to be the cause of Huntington's disease.

Task 2: Writing

For this part, you are allowed 30 minutes to write a composition on the topic: the current status of influenza prevention and control. You should write at least 120 words, and base your composition on the outline below:

1) Epidemic characteristics of influenza.

2) In the face of influenza virus mutation, what is the direction for vaccines and drugs?

Task 3: Oral Presentation

The struggle between humans and influenza viruses has been going on for many years. The emergence of vaccines and drugs has become a powerful tool for humans to fight against influenza. However, the cunning influenza viruses have gradually made vaccines and drugs ineffective through their own mutations. How can human beings completely defeat the flu virus in the future?

Learning Garden

The Birth of Smallpox Vaccine

Edward Jenner, a rural doctor in the UK, is a highly responsible physician. During the raging period of the smallpox virus, he vowed to find a safer and effective way to cure the terrible smallpox. Once, he discovered a strange phenomenon in a cattle farm: none of the milkmaids died of smallpox or turned into a pockmark.

In order to find out the reason, Jenner observed the cowshed many times afterwards and found that the milkmaid would indeed get cow smallpox. However, if one has cow smallpox, they only develop water sores between their fingers, experience a low-grade fever, and have localized lymph gland swelling, which will heal soon. Based on this observation, Jenner could preliminarily conclude that after an individual contracts cow smallpox, they be immune to smallpox. Beginning in 1788, Jenner continued his observations and experiments for eight years while conducting in-depth research on the symptoms of cow smallpox. From this extensive study, he concluded that vaccinia could prevent smallpox.

On May 21,1796, Jenner inoculated cowpox on a human for the first time. The recipient of the vaccination was an 8-year-old boy named Phipps. Jenner took some acne scars from a girl who had just been infected with smallpox and planted them on Phipps' left arm. For the first 3 days, Phipps felt a little uncomfortable but soon returned to normal, leaving only a faint scar where the vaccinia had grown. Six weeks later, Jenner exposed Phipps to the "pulp" of human smallpox. Since then, Phipps did not have any symptoms, indicating that the method of using vaccinia was effective and completely feasible. Since then, the cowpox method has spread all over the world, and the smallpox demon has finally been conquered by humans.

（孙力涛、孙彩军）

Unit 11   Health Economics and Health Management

READING A

PREVIEW

At the core of health economics and management is the idea to improve the efficiency, quality, and equity of the healthcare system by optimizing resource allocation under constrained budgets. Before the 2000s, the healthcare system in China was administratively cumbersome and organizationally outdated, thereby failing to adapt to the ever-increasing medical needs of its population. Since the early 2000s, major reforms have been undertaken to improve both healthcare financing and health services. These reforms have substantially changed the landscape of health insurance and medical facilities in China while visibly improving patient experience.

Questions for discussion

Q1: What were the foremost issues of the healthcare system in China since the 1980s?

Q2: What changes have been made to the health insurance schemes since 2003?

Text A

Background of the Healthcare Sector in China

During the early decades after 1949, community healthcare facilities were instrumental in securing access to medical attention in China. However, the importance of community healthcare facilities declined substantially from the 1980s to the 2000s in China. Inherited from the period of planned economy, the healthcare system in China during the 1980s was characterized by **bureaucracy** and centralization, which concentrated resources in large public hospitals. During this period, about 90% of both outpatient and inpatient services were provided by public hospitals. Among these, the vast majority of medical care was consumed in tertiary hospitals with more than 500 beds. Due to an almost complete absence of hospital service gatekeepers, it was not uncommon that tertiary hospitals had to offer basic primary care along with advanced services and research activities. On top of this, the general population's skepticism towards community healthcare facilities exacerbated such centralization. Public hospitals were largely overburdened by this extensive list of responsibilities, thereby causing substantial inefficiency of the healthcare system. In the meantime, China has been transitioning away from a planned economy since the early 1980s. As such, **fiscal** subsidies to community healthcare facilities were withdrawn or substantially reduced. In the wake of such **institutional** changes, community healthcare facilities suffered severe downsizing.

A defining moment for the reforms of the outdated healthcare system was the 2003 SARS (severe acute respiratory syndrome virus) outbreak. This outbreak was a wake-up call to overhaul the Chinese healthcare services by triggering wide-spread discontent with the already unpopular system. In response to this outbreak, the central government **deployed** a wave of health reforms starting with pilot programs in selected provinces, which were later expanded nationwide in 2009. Based on the 2009 State Council's health reform roadmap, policies to reform the system focused on five major areas. Namely, they were 1) universal basic medical insurance coverage; 2) the essential drug system; 3) primary health care service provision; 4) equitable public health services; and 5) public hospital improvements. During the implementation process of the initial reforming plan, the five areas were further filtered to three. Specifically, universal health insurance coverage, drug pricing, and public hospitals became the three pillars of the new system. In what follows, the reforms in the health insurance area were reviewed.

Health Insurance Reforms and Their Impacts

Before the 2003 reforms, the supply side of the healthcare sector in China was highly centralized, closely resembling the administrative sector. Due to the disproportionate responsibility of public hospitals, healthcare financing also directly centered on the supply side. Specifically, government funding directly went to the public providers instead of subsidizing the demand side, leading to a mismatch of resources between providers and the patients. In the meantime, along with economic development, there has been a substantial evolution in the disease burden spectrum which drove the rapid increases in expenditure on chronic and non-communicable diseases. Consequently, patient out-of-pocket (OOP) costs also rocketed. In the early 2000s, OOP contributions to healthcare expenditure peaked at about 60%, whereas government financing accounted for a mere 20%.

Although the government attempted to contain costs by putting caps on the unit prices of services and products, such efforts have failed to meet the expectations of the policymakers. In light of this, reforms since 2003 aimed to shift the system towards financing the demand side through the establishment of national-level basic medical insurance schemes, funded by both the government and society. The reforms relied on two approaches: expanding insurance coverage and redesigning payment mechanisms for healthcare providers. By implementing these reforms, it was expected that the new system could reduce out-of-pocket expenses for patients through risk sharing and discouraging low-value care without compromising quality.

Insurance Policy Setting

To lift OOP-related access barriers through robust healthcare financing, the central government has developed a system of universal medical insurance with three major insurance schemes: Urban Employee Basic Medical Insurance (Urban Employee Insurance) covering individuals employed in the formal sector in cities; Urban Resident Basic Medical Insurance (Urban Resident Insurance) for urban residents who had census registry (Hukou) in cities or towns but were unemployed or were working in the informal sector; and New Rural Cooperative Medical Insurance (Rural Resident Insurance) for rural residents. The Urban Employee Insurance program provides the most comprehensive benefit package. It includes cost-sharing co-payments for both inpatient and outpatient services. Also, **premiums** of the Urban Employee program are set in accordance with income level. In addition, the employers are requested to pay a portion of the premiums. Unlike the mandatory Urban Employee program for people with payrolls, Urban Resident and Rural Resident Insurances are both voluntary programs in which premiums are highly subsidized by the government. Both resident programs were characterized by relatively less generous benefits. In terms of covered services, the Urban Employee Insurance program is most extensive for both inpatient and outpatient care, whereas both Urban and Rural Resident Insurance cover primarily inpatient care and very limited outpatient services for selected chronic conditions. Since 2009, a national reimbursement drug list included 2,349 medicines and put these products under price regulation. The national reimbursement drug list has been updated annually since 2017.

Words and Expressions

bureaucracy   官僚体制

*An effective **bureaucracy** is important for public service delivery.*

fiscal   财政的；国库的

*That traditional **fiscal** constitution was no longer sustainable in 1997.*

institutional   制度性的；习惯性的

*Gender bias and **institutional** barriers can contribute to disparities between women and men.*

deploy   部署

*The government will **deploy** more than 200 law enforcement personnel to the border.*

premium   会员费；保险费

*In addition to your **premium**, you usually have to pay other costs for your health care.*

Language Points

medical attention   医疗处理

If a patient needs medical attention, it means the person needs help from a medical professional. The term "medical attention" is a synonym to "medical care".

*After the car accident, the driver was taken to the hospital to receive immediate **medical attention** for his injuries.*

out-of-pocket costs   自付费用

Out-of-pocket costs are the difference between the amount the healthcare provider charges for a medical service and what your health insurer pays.

*Despite having health insurance, the patient still had to pay significant **out-of-pocket costs** for the prescription medication that was not fully covered by their plan.*

risk sharing　风险共担

Health insurance is essentially a risk sharing arrangement in which risks of individuals are pooled.

*The new health insurance plan includes a **risk sharing** component, which means that the insurance company and the policyholder will share the cost of any unexpected medical expenses.*

EXERCISES

Task 1: Vocabulary Application

Fill in the blanks with the words given below. Change the form where necessary.

> scheme; bureaucracy; exacerbate; subsidize; reimbursement; overburden; inefficiency; discontent; spectrum; expenditure

1. _____ in healthcare organizations may be detrimental to the efficiency of doctors.

2. The medical security system in China mainly consists of three _____ that cover urban employees, urban residents, and rural residents.

3. Misalignment between incentives for the providers and the goals of the payers can severely _____ the already highlighted issue of overtreatment.

4. The last two decades have seen an accelerated effort to _____ private health insurance plans.

5. This report reviews and analyses different _____ policies for medicines applied by countries in the WHO European region.

6. Public hospitals were largely _____ by this extensive list of responsibilities, thereby causing substantial _____ of the healthcare system.

7. This outbreak was a wake-up call to overhaul the Chinese healthcare services by triggering wide-spread _____ with the already unpopular system.

8. The disease burden _____ has evolved substantially along with economic development, which drove the rapid increase of _____ on chronic and non-communicable diseases.

Task 2: Writing

For this part, you are allowed 30 minutes to write a composition on the topic: healthcare system. You should write at least 120 words, and base your composition on the outline below:

1) Community medicine and primary care are important for healthcare access.

2) Should the government finance healthcare facilities or patients?

3) Do you think there is disparity in healthcare resource utilization across formally employed individuals and the rest of the population?

Task 3: Oral Presentation

Health insurance was almost non-existent over a century ago. Try to explain why it is essential today and give us an example.

READING B

PREVIEW

An ideal primary health care system should provide people with essential health care, including basic public health services and clinical care, and meet most of their health needs within a community throughout their lifetime. A well-organized primary health care system can substantially improve the population's health welfare. Therefore, enhancing the primary health care system in China became one of the core intentions of the new round of health reform in 2009. With the implementation of the 2009 health reform, access to and affordability of primary health care have considerably improved, while the quality of primary health care remains of great concern in China. Understanding these challenges and finding the corresponding solutions are significant in building a strong primary health care system with good quality in China.

Questions for Discussion

Q1: What are the demanding challenges in China's primary health care system?

Q2: How can the quality of primary health care in China be improved?

Text B

Build a Strong Primary Health Care System with Good Quality of Care in China

"All people, everywhere, deserve the right care, right in their community." This is the fundamental **premise** of primary health care (PHC) **asserted** by the World Health Organization (WHO). PHC is defined as the essential health care based on scientifically sound and socially acceptable methods and technology, which should be able to address most of a person's health needs within a community throughout his/her lifetime. The ideal model of PHC was proposed by the WHO in the Declaration of Alma-Ata in 1978, which indicated that PHC activities should encompass health promotion, disease prevention, treatment, **rehabilitation** and **palliative** care as a whole-of-society approach. The WHO **elaborates** the main goals of PHC as the following three categories: satisfying people's health needs throughout their life, dealing with the determinants of health through multisectoral actions, and empowering people to be in charge of their own health.

The assessment of a PHC system could be based on three dimensions: quality, efficiency, and equity. Quality of care means the degree to which health services increase the likelihood of desired health outcomes. Efficiency of care means that health outcomes cannot be increased by reallocating the fixed amount of healthcare resources. And equity of care means that the quality of provided healthcare does not depend on personal characteristics such as gender, ethnicity, geographic location, and socioeconomic status. Among these three dimensions, quality is given priority because it is essential for improving health, which is the **ultimate** goal of a health system. Therefore, the assessment of quality is the focus in this article.

Regarding the PHC system in China, it is important to first review its history. China's PHC system was established in the early 1950s with the aim of providing universally **accessible** basic clinical care and public health services to people. At that time, the three-level network of the PHC system consisted of counties, communes and production brigades. During its early decades, the PHC system had performed well in reducing the burden of communicable, maternal, and neonatal diseases and received high praise from WHO.

However, in the decades following 1978, which marked the beginning of reform and opening-up, the PHC system faced challenges arising from market-based reforms in healthcare. These challenges included inadequate government health financing, **surging** medical costs, **diminishing** access to primary care facilities, widening regional inequities, and an **erosion** of healthcare workforce. A comprehensive health reform was in urgent need.

In response, China initiated a new round of health reform in 2009, one of the intentions of which was to enhance the PHC system. With the implementation of the 2009 health reform, access to and affordability of PHC have substantially improved, which can be **attributed** to increased government health financing, efforts towards achieving universal health coverage, the **initiation** of the basic public health service program, and the establishment of an essential drug system. Nevertheless, the quality of PHC remains of great concern in China.

Based on the assessment framework of the European Primary Care Monitoring System and considering the increasing prevalence of non-communicable diseases as well as the gatekeeping function pursued by PHC in China, three measures have been selected to assess the quality of PHC in China: quality of diagnosis and treatment, prescribing behavior, and quality of chronic disease management.

First, the quality of diagnosis and treatment at PHC facilities is evaluated as low. A survey conducted in the western region of China showed that PHC providers addressed only 36% of the essential questions or necessary examinations, and correctly diagnosed 26% of illnesses. Another survey conducted on patients with symptoms of classic pulmonary tuberculosis showed significant variation in doctors' behavior across different regions.

Second, concerning the prescribing behavior, the phenomenon of overusing antibiotics exists at PHC facilities. According to the recommendation by WHO, the average proportion of antibiotic use at PHC facilities should not be higher than 30%. However, systematic reviews have revealed that this proportion in China has reached 50%, with many prescriptions being **deemed** inappropriate.

Third, the ability of chronic disease management is weak in PHC settings in China. Hypertension and diabetes are the two most commonly treated chronic diseases at PHC facilities. According to some nationally representative surveys on hypertension, the awareness rates for hypertension and diabetes were 32% and 47%, **respectively**, and the control rates were even lower at 10% and 15%, respectively. This means that a patient diagnosed with hypertension through population screening (which is public health service) may not receive subsequent necessary treatment in a clinical sector. This reveals a significant gap between public health and clinical care, as well as their poor integration within PHC institutions. A similar phenomenon was observed in a nationwide longitudinal survey regarding diabetes.

According to the above assessments, the quality of PHC in China still needs to be improved. Drawing on the available literature, four challenges can be identified in the PHC system in China: **workforce** development, **remuneration** system and income of PHC **practitioners**, coordination of care, and continuity of care.

Firstly, PHC facilities face a shortage of qualified **professionals**, such as physicians, nurses, and public health practitioners. In 2010, 41% of PHC physicians in community health centers and 60% in township health centers had an education level lower than that of a junior medical college (**equivalent** to a licensed assistant physician). In 2011, the nationwide reform of graduate medical education was initiated, and training for family doctors was given priority. With the enacting of this policy, the number of qualified family doctors in PHC sectors has **dramatically** increased. By 2018, the percentage of professionals in community health centers and in township health centers with the level of education less than junior medical college decreased to 25% and 42%, respectively. Nevertheless, these figures are still higher than those observed in other high-income countries.

In addition, the income of PHC practitioners is primarily determined by the quantity rather than the quality of care provided. Medications and diagnostic tests are charged at higher rates than their usual costs, while labor-intensive services such as consultations are charged at lower rates. Besides, more than half of the revenue of PHC institutions comes from medication sales, which greatly influences physicians' income. Such a fee schedule would result in inappropriate incentives for physicians' behaviors. For example, they tend to sell more medication and do more diagnostic tests, instead of improving the quality of care. This is not only a waste of medical resources, but also a damage to people's health and welfare.

Furthermore, the PHC facilities in China function suboptimally in coordinating care, which should include serving as **gatekeepers** in the **tiered** healthcare delivery system with bidirectional referral mechanisms, and coordinating basic public health services and clinical care within the PHC settings. On the one hand, the establishment of gatekeepers is hindered by several factors. First, hospitals and PHC facilities have to compete for patients in order to increase revenues, resulting in no **incentives** to refer patients. Second, patients have the freedom to select between PHC facilities and hospitals for their initial doctor contact without any restrictions on reimbursement though without referral. Third, the electronic records for patients are not integrated between PHC facilities and hospitals. On the other hand, the provision of clinical care and public health services are not well combined due to two reasons. First, **financing** sources for these two kinds of care are different; public health is directly financed by the government while clinical care is paid by either the social health insurance or patients' **out-of-pocket** payment. Second, there is little information sharing or interaction between these two kinds of care delivery, though they happened in the same settings.

Last but not least, continuity of care is often neglected in PHC settings, which should **entail** the following three dimensions. First, patients' relational continuity with family doctors is important for patients' health. Therefore, the government has enacted a family doctor registration policy as the first step towards building a gatekeeping system. Second, informational continuity is inadequate since the electronic medical record system in PHC facilities are often unavailable or fragmented. Third, barriers exist in managerial continuity because PHC facilities and hospitals are financed and administered by different public sectors.

To tackle the challenges in improving the quality of PHC in China, the following policy recommendations could be considered.

First, the quality of training for professionals should be enhanced. The Ministry of Education should establish accreditation systems for physicians receiving **in-service** training. The government could also set goals for medical colleges about the percentage of graduates who continue with the postgraduate training. Additionally, academic discipline and practice guidelines should be **tailored** for PHC settings.

Second, a national performance assessment of PHC facilities should be conducted, and performance outcomes should be linked with incentives, such as physicians' income. PHC providers that perform well and provide high-quality care should be rewarded by increasing their payment from the social health insurance.

Moreover, the public health budget should be combined with the social health insurance budget, and the original payment method of **fee-for-service** should be replaced by a capitation payment method. Additionally, the amount of **capitation** payment should be adjusted for risk factors such as age and income. The adoption of the capitation payment method would help with the orientation changing for PHC practitioners from increasing the quantity of care to improving the quality of care.

Further, the coordination between PHC facilities and hospitals should be strengthened. In addition to simple technical support from hospitals to PHC facilities, deeper coordination is required between the two sectors. As proposed by the State Council of the People's Republic of China and practiced in other countries, a medical alliance or integrated delivery system should be established. Within such a system, special attention should be given to the allocation of economic interests and the design of payment mechanisms.

Finally, information systems should be improved. Within PHC facilities, a unified electronic health record system should be established by integrating the current Residents Health Record System for basic public health services and the Electronic Medical Record System for clinical care at PHC facilities. And such an information system should be available even in village clinics. Between PHC **facilities** and hospitals, such an information system should be linked with the information system adopted by **secondary** and **tertiary** hospitals.

As a conclusion, though China has made great achievements during the past decade since the new health reform in 2009, the quality of PHC is suboptimal and many challenges still exist in establishing a robust PHC system. It is hoped that by implementing appropriate measures, China can establish a strong PHC system with high-quality care.

Words and Expressions

premise 前提

*You should check the basic **premise** before drawing the conclusion.*

assert 声称；断言

*The factory **asserts** that the waste will not pollute the river.*

rehabilitation 康复；恢复

*A patient who has just recovered from a stroke may need **rehabilitation** to handle independently daily activities such as dressing or bathing.*

palliative 缓和的；姑息的

*The only feasible treatment for the elderly with deadly tumors is **palliative**.*

elaborate 详尽阐述

*The president resigned but refused to **elaborate** on the reason.*

ultimate 最后的；最终的

*The **ultimate** responsibility for the failure lies with the manager.*

accessible 可及的

*The hospital is easily **accessible** by road.*

surge 飞涨；激增

*Sales of the company have **surged** since the last recession.*

diminish 减少；降低

*The threat of the pandemic is **diminishing**.*

erosion 削弱；腐蚀；减少

*The survey reveals a gradual **erosion** of the army's support.*

attribute 把……归因于

*The lawyer **attributes** his success to lots of hard work.*

initiation 开始；发起

*The **initiation** of such a project is absolutely necessary.*

deem 认为；视为

*It is **deemed** to be impolite in some cultures if you stand too close to others.*

respectively 分别地；依次为

*She got an M.S. and a Ph.D. from Tsinghua University in 2000 and 2003 **respectively**.*

workforce 劳动力；全体员工

*Much of the **workforce** in this industry has been affected by the new policy.*

remuneration 酬金；薪水

*The government provides adequate **remuneration** for part-time employees.*

practitioner 专业人员；专门人才

*Dr. Wu is a general **practitioner** in the community health center.*

professional 专门人员；专业人士

*Doctors must learn how to interact with patients and also other health **professionals**.*

equivalent 相等的；相同的

*Every couple who has a third kid can be awarded a voucher **equivalent** to the money that would be spent on educating their child.*

dramatically 戏剧性地；显著地

*The great recession has **dramatically** affected the economy of the whole country.*

gatekeeper 守门人；把关系统

*The primary health care sectors act as **gatekeepers** who determine whether to refer patients to higher-level hospitals.*

tiered 分层的

This roasted turkey was served on tiered platters on this special Thanksgiving Day.

incentive 激励；刺激

*Tax **incentives** have been demonstrated to be effective in encouraging the investment.*

financing 提供资金；筹资

*The government has increased the percentage of **financing** for this project.*

out-of-pocket （费用）自掏腰包垫付的

*A health system is unfair if the **out-of-pocket** payment accounts for too large a proportion of the total health expenses.*

entail 涉及；牵涉

*The investment in the stock market would inevitably **entail** some risk.*

in-service 在职进行的；不脱产的

*The company provides its employees once **in-service** training each year.*

tailor 专门制作；定做

*We **tailor** our products to meet all the specific needs of our customers.*

fee-for-service 按项目支付医疗费

*The traditional **fee-for-service** payment is unfair since it cannot be adjusted according to patients' income.*

capitation 按人头付费

*Physicians in primary care facilities receive a **capitation** of 99.5RMB per patient.*

facility （供特定用途的）场所

*Maintaining hygiene is vital for health **facilities**.*

secondary 次要的；第二级的

*This **secondary** hospital is owned by the government.*

tertiary 第三位的；第三级的

*A **tertiary** hospital should not only provide medical services, but also educate medical students.*

Language Point

health need 健康需要

the minimum number of resources required to exhaust an individual's or a specified population's capacity to benefit from a health intervention

Health need is different with health demand (健康需求). Health need refers to the care that doctors believe is essential for a person to stay healthy but patients may not consume it due to subjective or financial reasons, while health demand may not be necessary but requires people to afford and be willing to pay for the medical cost.

*Inappropriate incentives would arouse excessive unnecessary **health demands**, while many*

*necessary **health needs**, meanwhile, cannot be fully met.*

determinants of health   健康决定因素

the range of personal, social, economic, and environmental factors that influence health status

*Social **determinants of health** can also affect a wide range of health outcomes.*

health promotion   健康促进

the process of enabling people to increase control over, and to improve their health, which is beyond the focus on individual behavior towards a wide range of social and environmental interventions

***Health promotion** is a money-saving way to improve the population's health status.*

give priority   优先考虑

to deal with or do (something) first

*The vulnerable group should be **given priority** when health resources are allocated.*

universal health coverage   全民健康覆盖

It means that all people have access to the health services they need, when and where they need them, without financial hardship.

***Universal health coverage** should be based on a strong primary health care system.*

community health center   社区卫生服务中心

a primary health care sector in the urban areas in China

*It is very convenient to visit my family doctor since the **community health center** lies only one block away.*

township health center   乡镇卫生院

a primary health care sector in the rural areas in China

*The majority of the Chinese rural population receive outpatient care in **township health centers***.

bidirectional referral   双向转诊

A bidirectional referral system is an organized two-way relationship between primary care providers and higher-level hospitals.

*China has made great efforts in building an effective **bidirectional referral** system.*

medical alliance   医联体

an integrated healthcare delivery system, where the provision of medical services by primary health care sectors and hospitals should be organized

*The establishment of **medical alliances** has been given priority in the past decade, which is believed to solve the current problems such as the high cost of medical care.*

EXERCISES

Task 1: Vocabulary Application

Fill in the blanks with the words given below. Change the form where necessary.

capitation; workforce; affordability; 3-tier; attribute; dramatically; deem; secondary; initiation; remuneration; tertiary; accessibility; fee-for-service; facility; gatekeeper

1. Hospitals in China have been classified in a _____ system, including the primary health care _____ , _____ hospitals, and _____ hospitals.

2. The mayor asked the committee to take whatever steps he _____ necessary to recover the economy of the city.

3. The _____ of the New Cooperative Medical Scheme improved _____ the _____ and the _____ of health care in rural China.

4. Different payment methods have different shortages. For instance, the _____ payment tends to incentivize physicians to prescribe more than needed, while the _____ payment may encourage physicians to cut necessary treatment since health insurance sectors can only pay hospitals a fixed amount of fee per patient.

5. The rapid social development should be partially _____ to the new technology.

Task 2: Writing

"What is the current status of the primary health care system in China? What is the most demanding challenge in functioning as gatekeepers in your opinion?" This is a question posted by a user on a social question-and-answer website. Please write an answer to this post. You should write at least 150 words but no more than 300 words.

Task 3: Oral Presentation

The development of Chinese primary health care system is facing great challenges. The ministry of health is collecting suggestions from the public on how to improve the provision of primary health care in China. And you have been appointed as the representative for students. Please prepare an 8-minute presentation and provide your opinions concerning the above issue.

Learning Garden

The Declaration of Alma-Ata in 1978

Under the coordination of the World Health Organization and the United Nations International Children's Emergency Fund, the International Conference on Primary Health Care was held in Alma-Ata, the capital city of Former Soviet Kazakh Republic in 1978. This conference was inspired by China's barefoot doctor system, based on which the Declaration of Alma-Ata, as a major milestone of the twentieth century in the field of public health, was put forward. The concept of primary health care was first proposed in this declaration and was identified as the key to the attainment of the goal of Health for All. This declaration expressed the need for urgent actions by all governments, health professionals, and the world community to promote health for all the people in the world.

（蒋亚文、徐明明）

Reference

[1] LI X, LU J, HU S, et al. The primary health-care system in China[J]. Lancet, 2017, 390(10112):2584-2594.

[2] LI X, KRUMHOLZ H M, YIP W, et al. Quality of primary health care in China: challenges and recommendations[J]. Lancet, 2020, 395(10239):1802-1812.

Unit 12   Evidence-Based Medicine and Systematic Review

READING A

PREVIEW

*In response to limitations in understanding and using published evidence, evidence-based medicine (EBM) emerged as a movement in the early 1990s. Initially, EBM focused on educating clinicians about understanding and using published literature to **optimize** clinical care, including the science of systematic reviews. EBM progressed to recognize limitations of evidence alone, and has increasingly stressed the need to combine critical **appraisal** of the evidence with patient's values and preferences through shared decision making. In another progress, EBM incorporated and further developed the science of producing trustworthy clinical practice guidelines **pioneered** by investigators in the 1980s. EBM's enduring contributions to clinical medicine include placing the practice of medicine on a solid scientific basis, the development of more **sophisticated** **hierarchies** of evidence, the recognition of the crucial role of patient values and preferences in clinical decision making, and the development of the methodology for generating trustworthy recommendations.*

Task 1: Questions for Discussion

Q1: What is evidence-based medicine?

Q2: How do we achieve real evidence-based medicine?

Text A

Return to Real Evidence-based Medicine

Since the time of Hippocrates, medicine has struggled to balance the uncontrolled experience of healers with observations obtained by **rigorous** investigation of claims regarding the effects of health interventions. During the past 300 years, demands that the practice of medicine be founded on scientifically trustworthy **empirical** evidence have become increasingly vocal.

In the 1970s and 1980s, David Sackett, David Eddy, and Archie Cochrane (among others) highlighted the need for strengthening the empirical practice of medicine and proposed initial evidentiary rules for guiding clinical decisions. In 1991, Gordon H Guyatt introduced the term evidence-based medicine (EBM), with a focus on educating front-line clinicians in assessing the **credibility** of research evidence, understanding the results of clinical studies, and determining how best to apply the results to their everyday practice. Subsequently, detailed guidance published in journal articles and associated textbooks, complemented by popular tools such as the Graphic Appraisal Tool for Epidemiology, resulted in EBM becoming increasingly **integrated** into medical curricula worldwide. Additionally, ratings of important developments in medicine have placed EBM on par with antibiotics and anesthesia for the practice of medicine.

On the surface, EBM proposes a specific association between medical evidence, theory, and practice. EBM does not, however, offer a new scientific theory of medical knowledge, but instead has progressed as a coherent heuristic structure for optimizing the practice of medicine that explicitly and conscientiously attends to the nature of medical evidence. Central to the epistemology of EBM is that what is justifiable or reasonable to believe depends on the trustworthiness of the evidence, and the extent to which we believe that evidence is determined by credible processes. Although EBM acknowledges a role for all empirical observations, it contends that controlled clinical observations provide more trustworthy evidence than do uncontrolled observations, biological experiments, or individual clinician's experiences.

The basis for the first EBM **epistemological** principle is that not all evidence is created equal, and that the practice of medicine should be based on the best available evidence. The second principle endorses the philosophical view that the pursuit of truth is best accomplished by evaluating the totality of the evidence, and not selecting evidence that favors a particular claim. Evidence is, however, necessary but not sufficient for effective decision making, which has to address the consequences of importance to the decision maker within the given environment and context. Thus, the third epistemological principle of EBM is that clinical decision making requires consideration of patients' values and preferences.

The research agenda for real evidence-based medicine is much broader than critical appraisal and draws on a wider range of underpinning disciplines. For example, it should include the study of the patient's experiences of illness and the real-life clinical encounters in different conditions and circumstances. The field would be enriched, for example, by qualitative research to elucidate the logic of care–that is, the numerous elements of good illness management that are **complementary** to the application of research evidence.

We need to gain a better understanding (perhaps beginning with a **synthesis** of the cognitive psychology literature) of how clinicians and patients find, **interpret**, and evaluate evidence from research studies, and how (and if) these processes feed into clinical communication, exploration of diagnostic options, and shared decision making. Furthermore, it is necessary to conduct a more in-depth study on the less **algorithmic** components of the clinical method such as intuition and **heuristic** reasoning, and how evidence may be incorporated into such reasoning.

Scientific communities have embraced EBM-related initiatives to develop guidance and checklists for improving design, conduct, and reporting of research. Over the past 25 years, numerous such initiatives have occurred, including checklists and statements on how to develop a research protocol and report randomized trials, observational studies, diagnostic test studies, predictive models, and genetic testing studies; they can be accessed via the EQUATOR website. Alongside these developments, researchers have increasingly differentiated between explanatory (also known as mechanistic or proof-of-concept efficacy) trials that address the question "can intervention work in the ideal setting?" versus pragmatic (also known as practical, effectiveness) trials that address the question "does it work in real-world settings?" and "is it worth it and should it be paid for? (efficiency)".

There is some evidence suggesting that these initiatives have resulted in an improvement in the quality of research reporting; for instance, the reporting of RCTs has improved as a result of the CONSORT checklist. While optimal reporting is desirable, what's worse than poor reporting is the failure to report or suppression of clinical research. Currently, only 50% of trials conducted by investigators are reported, posing a significant and avoidable threat to the body of scientific knowledge. When half of studies are unreported, both patient care and new research initiatives will often suffer from flaws. Despite long-standing awareness of publication bias as a problem, the only possible solution- registration of all trial protocols before research is actually undertaken, and full reporting of the results in a timely manner after the study is completed- received only haphazard adherence in 2016.

In relation to producing usable evidence, we need to identify how to balance gold-standard systematic reviews with pragmatic, rapid reviews that gain in timeliness and accessibility which they lose in-depth and detail. In the same vein, we need research on how and in what circumstances to trade detail for brevity in developing guidelines. We need to develop decision aids that support clinicians and patients to clarify the goals of care, raise and answer questions about the quality and completeness of evidence, and understand and **contextualize** estimates of benefit and harm. We also need to improve both the usefulness and ease-of-use of these and other evidence-based tools (models, scores, algorithms, and so on) including the intellectual, social, and **temporal** demands they make on users and the resource implications for the healthcare organization and system.

In relation to effectiveness, we need greater attention to post marketing research in day-to-day hospital and primary care settings to confirm that subsequent experience **replicates** the results of licensing trials. This will allow for the revision of gold standard tests and their cut-off points for ruling out diagnoses and treatments, aiming to minimize overdiagnosis or underdiagnosis.

Finally, in relation to the collective effort to prevent the misappropriation of the evidence-based quality mark, a key research priority remains studying hidden biases in sponsored research, such as refining statistical techniques for challenging findings that appear too good to be true.

Much progress has been made and lives have been saved through the systematic collation, synthesis, and application of high-quality empirical evidence. However, evidence-based medicine has not resolved the problems it set out to address (especially evidence biases and the hidden hand of vested interests), which have become more subtle and harder to detect. Furthermore, contemporary healthcare's complex economic, political, technological, and commercial context has tended to steer the evidence-based agenda towards populations, statistics, risk assessment, and **spurious** certainty. Despite paying lip service to shared decision-making, patients can be left confused or even tyrannized when their clinical management is inappropriately driven by algorithmic protocols, top-down directives, and population targets.

Words and Expressions

optimize 使优化，完善

*As air breathing increased in importance, the vertebrate larynx strengthened to accommodate additional functions such as **optimizing** airflow and protecting the lungs from foreign matter.*

pioneer 先驱，先锋，创始人；做先锋，当开拓者，倡导

*No doubt happenstance bears much responsibility for the direction taken by an academic career, but there was another influence at work on our **pioneers**.*

sophisticated 精于世故的，老练的；见多识广的；很有品位的；精密的，复杂的；高级的

*A more **sophisticated** argument might be that, although a number of geometries are consistent with physical space, only one can be accommodated to physical theory.*

hierarchy 等级制度

*Without really challenging the **hierarchy**, they still squeezed concessions out of village leaders, thereby turning a weakness into strength.*

rigorous 严密的，缜密的；严谨的

*Indeed, most past work has focused on implementation issues; our current work focuses on defining **rigorous** semantics.*

empirical 以经验（或实验）为依据的；经验主义的；来自经验（或观察）的

*However, this venue of hyper-abstraction leads to immunity and removes internalization from the **empirical** discourse.*

credibility 可信性；可靠性

*What gives that claim its **credibility** is the fact that it does not overlook or gainsay the routineness of the routine cases.*

integrated 结合的；整合的；融合的

*Customers are looking for flexible **integrated** solutions to help them make better decisions faster.*

epistemological 认识论的

*However, before we present our data, there is another important methodological, indeed **epistemological**, issue.*

appraisal 评价

*The newspaper gave an editorial **appraisal** of the government's achievements of the past year.*

complementary 互补的

*My family and my job both play an important part in my life, fulfilling separate but **complementary** needs.*

synthesis 合成

*Biocatalysis plays an important role in the **synthesis** of complex organic molecules.*

interpret　解释

*It's difficult to **interpret** these statistics without knowing how they were obtained.*

algorithmic　算法的

*The software can in theory do anything you like as long as it is an **algorithmic** process.*

heuristic　（教学法）启发式的, 探索式的

*A bigger problem with the head mapping **heuristic** is that some answers referring to the same entity are not merged.*

contextualize　将……置于环境中

*It is not sufficient to merely reproduce narratives without **contextualizing** them within a larger social and political framework.*

temporal　世俗的

*The drug reduces spatial and **temporal** awareness.*

replicate　复制

*Researchers tried many times to **replicate** the original experiment.*

spurious　伪造的; 虚假的

*Some of the arguments in favor of shutting the factory are questionable and others are downright **spurious**.*

Language Points

evidence-based　循证的, 实证的, 以大量科研为基础的

An approach to medicine, education, and other disciplines that emphasizes the practical application of the findings of the best available current research, supported by a large amount of scientific research.

*Nowadays, the term "**evidence-based**" is used in numerous situations and conditions, such as **evidence-based** medicine, **evidence-based** practice, **evidence-based** health care, **evidence-based** social work, **evidence-based** policy, and **evidence-based** education. **Evidence-based** medicine (EBM) is the conscientious, explicit, and judicious use of current best evidence in making decisions regarding the care of individual patients. This concept has gained popularity recently, and its applications have been steadily expanding.*

EXERCISES

Task 1: Vocabulary Application

Fill in the blanks with the words given below. Change the form where necessary.

algorithmically; empirical; optimize; temporally; sophisticated; contextual; evidence-based; integrate; promote; contemporary

1. A major point we take from the many comments is a prevailing feeling in the research community that we need significantly and urgently to advance resilience research, both by

sharpening concepts and theories and by conducting _____ studies at a much larger scale and with a much more extended and _____ methodological arsenal than is the case currently.

2. The objective of this study is to determine if _____ generated double-booking recommendations could increase patient volume per clinical session without increasing the burden on physicians.

3. Field notes are widely recommended in qualitative research as a means of documenting needed _____ information.

4. Furthermore, we show that _____ mediated schematic knowledge biases reasoning decisions in an age-dependent manner.

5. Beyond application of best practice recommendations to guide safe use and _____ clinical outcome, several issues are better addressed through _____ policies, procedures, and practices.

6. When practiced effectively, EBM _____ clinical expertise, patients' values, and best evidence, and _____ optimal patient care.

7. Furthermore, _____ healthcare's complex economic, political, technological, and commercial context has tended to steer the evidence-based agenda towards populations, statistics, risk, and spurious certainty.

Task 2: Writing

For this part, you are allowed 30 minutes to write a composition on the topic of evidence-based medicine. You should write at least 120 words, and base your composition on the outline below:

1) Crisis in evidence-based medicine

2) The real evidence-based medicine

3) Actions to deliver real evidence-based medicine

Task 3: Oral Presentation

This era of groundbreaking scientific developments in high-resolution, high-throughput technologies allows for the cost-effective collection and analysis of vast and diverse datasets on individual health. This means that precision medicine needs to be contrasted with evidence-based medicine, a powerful and widely used practice informed by meta-analyses or group-centered studies from which mean recommendations are derived. Combining knowledge about evidence-based medicine, try to describe the possible bridge between precision medicine and evidence-based medicine.

READING B

PREVIEW

*Systematic reviews are fundamental to evidence-based healthcare and provide the highest level of evidence for decision making. Meta-analysis is a quantitative **synthesis** of information from systematic reviews, which statistically combines results from multiple studies to make the* *best use of available evidence. It has become increasingly important in recent decades as the need for a robust evidence base has become apparent in many scientific areas, including medicine and health, social sciences, education, psychology, ecology, and economics.*

Task 1: Questions for Discussion

Q1: What is the relationship between systematic review and meta-analysis?

Q2: What are the advantages and disadvantages of meta-analysis?

Text B

Systematic Reviews and Meta-analysis: Synthesis of Evidence for Decision making

Systematic Review and Meta-analysis

Systematic reviews are fundamental to evidence-based healthcare and provide the highest level of evidence for decision making. The role of systematic reviews in healthcare has evolved to acknowledge the **overwhelming** amount of available research evidence. A systematic review involves a structured literature search to combine information from studies, using a pre-designed protocol, aiming to address a specific research question. The process aims to find and use all available published and unpublished evidence, carefully evaluate it, and objectively summarize it to reach **defensible** recommendations. The synthesis of information can be **qualitative** or quantitative.

A qualitative synthesis typically summarizes the scientific and methodological characteristics of the included studies (e.g., size, population, interventions, quality of **execution**); the strengths and limitations of their design and execution and the effect of these factors on study conclusions; their relevance to the populations, comparisons, settings, and outcomes or measures of interest defined by the research questions; and patterns in the relationships between study characteristics and study outcomes. Such qualitative summaries help answer questions that are not **amenable** to statistical analysis.

A meta-analysis is a quantitative synthesis of information from a systematic review. Statistical analyses are employed to summarize outcomes across studies, using either **aggregate**d summary data from trial reports or complete data from individual participants. When comparing the effectiveness and safety of treatments between groups of individuals who receive different treatments or exposures, meta-analysis summarizes the differences as treatment effects, with the size and corresponding uncertainty estimates expressed using standard **metrics that** depend on the scale of the outcome being measured, such as continuous, categorical, count, or time-to-event variables. When the aim of the analysis is not to compare treatments, summaries may take the form of means or proportions of a single group.

Questions Addressed by Meta-analysis

In general, meta-analysis is used to address four types of questions. The first type is descriptive, summarizing some characteristic of a distribution, such as the prevalence of a disease, the mean of a population characteristic, or the sensitivity of a diagnostic test. For example, the awareness of HIV pre-exposure prophylaxis (PrEP) and willingness to use HIV PrEP among men who have sex with men (MSM) can be summarized to provide **implications** for HIV prevention in high-incidence groups. The sensitivity and specificity of HIV rapid testing could be collected to calculate pooled estimates, which can facilitate the generation of evidence for policy recommendations.

The second type of question is comparative, which is the most common. How does one treatment (e.g., vitamin D supplementation) compare with another (placebo) in reducing the risk of total cancer mortality? Does the new treatment **confer** significant benefits compared with the conventional treatment? Some of these questions relate to specific interventions, others relate to prevalent exposures, and others relate to diagnostic tests. When there are more than two treatments, a network meta-analysis (NMA) can be performed for comparing all pairs of treatments and ranking them by outcomes. NMA **aspires** to synthesize evidence about multiple treatments using valid statistical methods and can provide a broader picture of the available treatment options for a condition, identify research gaps, create a treatment hierarchy, and inform healthcare decision making.

A third type of question involves non-comparative associations, such as correlations between outcomes or the structure of an underlying pathway, and associations between variables in a regression model (e.g., dose-response relationships). For example, suppose you want to evaluate whether the relationship between self-confidence and sport performance, adjusted for the effects of cognitive and **somatic** anxiety, is stronger in individual sports than in team sports. On the one hand, under a univariate framework, the researcher would directly extract partial effect sizes from the primary studies and compare those from team sports and individual sports. On the other hand, under a multivariate framework, the researcher would extract correlation **matrices** and sport type from the studies. Then they would separate the team and individual sport studies to compute mean r matrices and path models or partial effect sizes for each subset.

A fourth type of question involves developing a prognostic or predictive model for an outcome. Prediction models are increasingly common in the literature, aiming to provide estimates of absolute risk of an outcome. Individualized risk predictions are provided to support decision making and can be improved by combining information from different data sources or published models using meta-analysis techniques.

How to Perform a Meta-analysis

The procedures for conducting a meta-analysis are as follows. First, prepare a research question forming the basis of a meta-analysis. Second, search the relevant literature using a variety of sources to address the research question. Third, extract relevant data from each study included in the analysis. Fourth, appraise the included studies and assess risk of bias critically. Fifth, assess the **heterogeneity** of the results to determine whether variations among the studies indicate real differences in the estimated effect or are merely due to sampling error. The Cochran's Q and I^2 statistics are usually used to test for heterogeneity. For the Q statistic, a P value greater than 0.10 suggests no significant heterogeneity. I^2 values range from 0% to 100%, with values of 25%, 50%, and 75% being interpreted as small, moderate, and high levels of heterogeneity, respectively. If heterogeneity is absent, a fixed-effects model is used to calculate a pooled estimate of the effect by taking a weighted average of all studies, along with a confidence interval that demonstrates the precision of this point estimate. Otherwise, if heterogeneity exists, a random-effects model is employed. A high level of heterogeneity does not necessarily indicate that a meta-analysis is incorrect, but such variation requires explanation. Meta-regression and subgroup analysis can be applied to investigate potential causes of the heterogeneity. Forest plots are usually used to graphically present the results of data synthesis. Other techniques and plots, such as sensitivity analysis and funnel plots, can be used to analyze and display patterns in the data. Sensitivity analysis involves repeating the analysis with alternative or different decisions than those originally made, allowing for an assessment of the robustness of the results to these different choices. Funnel plots and Egger's test are usually performed to test for publication bias.

The Preferred Reporting Items for Systematic Reviews and Meta-Analyses (PRISMA) statement is the primary guideline for reporting a meta-analysis of randomized studies. This statement lists 27 items that should be included in any report and are required by most journals that publish meta-analyses. These items include wording for the title as well as elements within the introduction, methods, results, and discussion sections. Slightly different requirements exist for observational studies which can be found in the Meta-analysis of Observational Studies in Epidemiology (MOOSE) statement. Additionally, several extensions of the PRISMA statement have been developed to facilitate reporting different types or aspects of meta-analyses such as those for individual participant data (PRISMA-IPD), networks of treatments (PRISMA-NMA), and diagnostic test accuracy (PRISMA-DTA).

Advantages of Meta-analysis

Meta-analysis provides a rational and helpful way of dealing with a number of practical difficulties that confront anyone attempting to comprehend effectiveness research. It provides an estimate of the average magnitude of a characteristic within a population, or the effectiveness or harm of a treatment (exposure), and an understanding of the variation in these quantities across different study settings. If the variation is not significant or can be comprehended, meta-analysis can increase the generalizability of research findings and determine their effects in subgroups. The unsystematic (or narrative) reviews include only a subset of relevant studies, which may introduce bias. Certain reports that are potentially favorable may be more likely to be included in a review than those without any significant differences. In addition, informal synthesis may be **tainted** by the prior beliefs of the reviewer. However, conducting a meta-analysis on a rigorous systematic review can address these issues found in narrative reviews and provide an impartial synthesis of empirical data. By combining small studies, meta-analysis can also increase the precision with which key parameters are estimated and help to explain inconsistent results that occur when underpowered studies report non-statistically significant conclusions due to insufficient sample sizes. Meta-analysis can also focus on **discrepancies** in study results that might argue against combining their results, or might argue for more **subtle** interpretations of parameters whose true values might vary with characteristics of the populations studied or with the way in which interventions are undertaken. In some cases, exploring the causes of such heterogeneity may lead to important conclusions in their own right or may indicate the need for further studies to fill in research gaps.

Disadvantages of Meta-analysis

Although meta-analysis is a powerful technique, as with all research methods, it must be used with caution. A common criticism is the use of "apples and oranges", meaning that the included studies are **superficially** similar but are actually different. Apples and oranges are both fruits, but they are quite different. Heterogeneity statistics can assess variations between study results, but not clinical or methodological disparities. While visually helpful, forest plots are **devoid** of contextual information and consequently may be misleading. For example, a meta-analysis on antibiotics for treating urinary tract infections would be meaningless without knowing the type of infection and the type of antibiotic used in each study. Merely looking at the forest plot does not provide information about the duration of antibiotic regimen or other potential underlying conditions. Although these criticisms have some validity, the **transparency** of meta-analysis is its strength. Forest plots are a powerful way to present the results of studies, while meta-analyses should at least be transparent.

Another criticism, "garbage in, garbage out", is relatively straightforward and refers to the importance of conducting a **thorough** search for articles. A meta-analysis is limited by the quality of the individual study and is only as good as the studies included in the analysis. Therefore, while collecting your data, it's not just about finding relevant articles but also critically evaluating them to ensure that they meet your standards. Consequently, a meaningful meta-analysis should be performed within the framework of systematic reviews, using a systematic approach to minimize bias and address the combinability of studies.

Conclusions

Meta-analyses provide a systematic and quantitative approach to synthesizing evidence in response to the focused questions for healthcare practitioners and policy makers. Nonetheless, the execution of meta-analyses is fraught with pitfalls, and is fundamentally limited by the quality of the included studies. For healthcare practitioners and policy makers, carefully reviewing of published meta-analyses and conducting a balanced appraisal of their deficiencies is likely to become an increasingly important way to resolve uncertainty for the focused questions.

Words and Expressions

synthesis （人工或物质在动植物体内的）合成, 综合, 结合, 综合体
*The purpose of this study is to conduct a realist **synthesis** of research on effective strategies to support implementation of public health interventions.*

overwhelming 势不可挡的, 压倒性的, 巨大的, 无法抗拒的; overwhelm 的现在分词, 压倒, （感情或感觉）充溢, 难以禁受, 击败, 征服, 压垮, 使应接不暇
*The evidence for rapid climate change now seems **overwhelming**.*

defensible 可辩解的, 合乎情理的, 有正当理由的, 可防御的, 可守护的
*Some of the estimates are more inclusive and therefore more **defensible** than others.*

qualitative 质量的, 定性的, 性质的
***Qualitative** research uses a variety of methods, such as intensive interviews or in-depth analysis*

of historical material, and is concerned with a comprehensive account of some event or unit.

execution　处决,实行,执行,实施,表演,(乐曲的)演奏,(艺术品的)制作,(尤指遗嘱的)执行

Significant efforts and financial support have been made to involve patients in the design and execution of medical research.

amenable　易控制的,顺从的,顺服的,可用某种方式处理的

A principal finding of this study is that mortality due to amenable causes dropped more than mortality from non-amenable causes for both sexes.

aggregate　总计,合计;总数,(混凝土或修路等用的)骨料,集料

We present a framework for aggregating the divergent health effects associated with various types of environmental exposure, such as air pollution, residential noise, and significant technological risks.

metric　米制的,公制的,按公制制作的,用公制测量的;度量标准,[数学]度量,诗体,韵文,诗韵

There are several different metrics that can be used to determine if a population is living longer over time, for example, the proportion of adults living with cystic fibrosis, death rate, age at death, median survival age, or life expectancy.

implication　可能的影响(或作用、结果),含意,暗指,(被)牵连、牵涉

In this nationwide study, we aimed to evaluate the prevalence of smoking and its implication on chronic diseases in the Chinese population.

confer　商讨,协商,交换意见,授予(奖项、学位、荣誉或权利)

Breastfeeding might confer protection against obesity later in life, but the evidence is inconclusive.

aspire　渴望(成就),有志(成为)

They have sought to address the challenge of how to motivate and inspire women to aspire towards leadership roles as a key strategic goal.

somatic　体细胞的,躯体的,体的,体壁的

The prevalence of emotional distress is substantially elevated in people with a chronic somatic illness.

matrices　matrix 的复数,矩阵,(人或社会成长发展的)社会环境,政治局势,线路网,道路网,基体,矩阵转接电路,杂基

Job-exposure matrices (JEM) are a common method of exposure assessment in occupational epidemiology.

heterogeneity　异质性,不均匀性,不纯一性,多相性,个别市场变异,异类混淆

Although the heterogeneity of primary tumors has long been known, we show here that early disseminated cancer cells are genomically very unstable as well.

taint　污点,玷污,污染,腐坏;使腐坏,败坏(名声)

My remarks are not intended to be definitive, and definitely have the taint of personal opinion.

discrepancy　差异,不符合,不一致

Weighting was used to adjust for these geographic and demographic discrepancies.

subtle　不易察觉的, 不明显的, 微妙的, 机智的, 机巧的, 狡猾的, 巧妙的, 敏锐的

The distinction between social anxiety disorder and generalized anxiety disorder can be **subtle** *when anxiety about social situations predominates.*

devoid　缺乏, 完全没有

The dormant state of bacterial spores is generally considered to be **devoid** *of biological activity.*

transparency　透明度, 透明, 透明性, 幻灯片, 透明正片, 显而易见, 一目了然, 易懂

Given its well-known commitment to social justice, the HIV research community should lead the way in addressing incentive **transparency**.

superficially　从表面上看

The length of the chapter limits the ability to go into great detail about specific treatments and only **superficially** *mentions attention to diet, exercise, and stress management.*

thorough　彻底的, 完全的, 深入的, 细致的, 仔细周到, 工作缜密, 十足的, 彻头彻尾的, 完完全全的

All parents should be offered a **thorough** *evaluation, including a high-quality autopsy and placental histopathology.*

pitfall　陷阱, 困难, 危险,（尤指）隐患

In this review, we discuss the process of accurately establishing the diagnosis of brain tumors, with a focus on common **pitfalls** *encountered in clinical practice.*

Language Point

narrative review　叙述性综述, 传统的文献综述

An umbrella term for a collection of review types in which the review process goes beyond an opinion or commentary, in which researchers can pursue an extensive description and interpretation of previously published writing on a chosen topic.

Traditionally, practitioners relied on experts to summarize the literature and make recommendations in articles that became known as **narrative reviews**.

garbage in, garbage out　无用输入, 无用输出

The idea that in any system, the quality of output is determined by the quality of the input. For example, if a mathematical equation is improperly stated, the answer is unlikely to be correct.

GIGO is short for **garbage in, garbage out**, *which is programmer slang for bad output caused by faulty data.*

EXERCISES

Task 1: Vocabulary Application
Fill in the blanks with the words given below. Change the form where necessary.

> overwhelming; defensible; qualitative; implication; heterogeneity; taint; thorough; discrepancy; transparency; pitfall

1. We used a descriptive analytic study design with quantitative and _____ data collected from records and individual feedback from patients and health care providers.

2. For public health interventions to result in sustainable change, they need to both be effective in addressing the health burden and be economically _____.

3. For global health programs, the _____ is that the family and network may also be in need of health interventions and are often influential in help seeking and adherence.

4. Like previous attempts, we encountered significant _____ that was not explained using a comprehensive meta-regression approach.

5. Suffering is the perception of serious threat or damage to the self, and it emerges when a _____ develops between what one expected of one's self and what one does or is.

6. These studies have been modest in size, largely retrospective, and without _____ prospective clinical validation.

7. Price_____ efforts by certain states and health plans have sought to provide more actionable price information by focusing on reimbursement from the insurer or the out-of-pocket costs paid by the patient.

8. Even in high-income countries, the cost of medical care and associated societal burdens of dementia threaten to become _____ as more people live into old age.

9. Nevertheless, this technology is still relatively new, so we would like to highlight the pearls and _____ for point-of-care ultrasound (POCUS) users to use this tool to its full potential and ensure optimal patient care and safety.

10. While observational studies can provide important data, a randomized trial will minimize biases that may _____ the results, such as patient characteristics or other confounding factors differing between treatment arms.

Task 2: Writing

Defining a research question is the first and most important step in conducting systematic reviews and meta-analyses. For this part, you are required to write an essay of at least 150 words on how to prepare a research question for a meta-analysis.

Task 3: Oral Presentation

For this part, please pick up a topic of your research interest to conduct a meta-analysis. You are given 8 minutes to present your research plan briefly. Alternatively, you can provide us with a brief overview of the protocol used in a published meta-analysis in your research field.

Learning Garden

Cochrane Library

The Cochrane Library (named after Archie Cochrane) is a collection of databases in medicine and other healthcare specialties provided by Cochrane and other organizations. At its core is the collection of Cochrane Reviews, a database of systematic reviews and meta-analyses which summarize and interpret the results of medical research. The aim of the Cochrane Library is to readily provide the results of well-conducted controlled trials, making it a key resource in evidence-based medicine.

The Cochrane Library consists of the following databases after significant changes in 2018:

1. The Cochrane Database of Systematic Reviews (Cochrane Reviews). Contains all the peer-reviewed systematic reviews and protocols (Cochrane Protocols) prepared by the Cochrane Review Groups.

2. The Cochrane Central Register of Controlled Trials (CENTRAL). CENTRAL is a database that contains details of articles on controlled trials and other studies of healthcare interventions from bibliographic databases (majorly MEDLINE and EMBASE), and other published and unpublished sources that are difficult to access, including trials from the trial registries such as International Clinical Trials Registry Platform (ICTRP) and ClinicalTrials.gov. However, systematic reviewers need to search not only CENTRAL but also ICTRP and ClinicalTrials.gov to identify unpublished studies.

3. Cochrane Clinical Answers. These evidence summaries on a variety of questions of interest to healthcare professionals have a user-friendly presentation with graphics and high-level conclusions of the research evidence based on Cochrane Reviews.

（江洪波、邹华春）